To Shoshana

MAKING

THE

GOLDEN YEARS GOLDEN

*Resources and Sources of Information to Guide You
in Making the Right Decisions for Living Better,
Healthier, Independently And Stress-Free.*

by

Eva Mor

authorHOUSE®

AuthorHouse™
1663 Liberty Drive, Suite 200
Bloomington, IN 47403
www.authorhouse.com
Phone: 1-800-839-8640

First published by AuthorHouse   3/4/2009

ISBN: 978-1-4389-3930-8 (sc)
ISBN: 978-1-4389-3931-5 (hc)

Library of Congress Control Number: 2008911530

Printed in the United States of America
Bloomington, Indiana

This book is printed on acid-free paper.

Book Editing:
Laura Schraub Siegel
Ethan J. Sacks
Danielle E. Mor

DEDICATION

In memory of my beloved father, Leib.
To my mother Anna, and all the elderly people like her,
I dedicate this book.

To Gabi, my beloved husband, my partner and
best friend, without whom this book would never come to be.

And to my children, Ethan, Danielle, my sweet
granddaughter Naomi, and adopted daughter Masako.
You are the joy and blessings of my life.

Your love and support is my life line.

DISCLAMER

This book does not intend to replace the services of your doctors and other health providers. Any changes to one's diet or physical activities should be cleared by one's personal physician who is familiar with one's health status.

Always practice safety measures and consult with the appropriate advisors. In this book I have tried to inform and educate regarding the different issues that relate to the life of the senior, but the final decision and responsibility is yours. It is not the intent of either the author or the publisher to provide medical, legal or financial services. Those services should be furnished by your doctors, lawyer, or financial adviser. The author and the publisher disclaim any liability, loss or risk, personal or otherwise, resulting as a direct or indirect consequence from the reader's use or application of any of the contents of this book.

Every time a real person's story has been told, all names and identifying details have been changed to protect the privacy of the person and their family.

Contents

INTRODUCTION

Watching my parents age has been quite disheartening, their illnesses slowly eating away at their ability to do simple things that are taken for granted by all of us. I have worked most of my adult life with the elderly and the disabled, and was quite unprepared to deal with the emotional connotations of my parents' situation. This brought me to the subject of how to improve my parents' daily life, prolong it, and enrich it.

In the last 23 years I have worked in the health-related field. I have worked in hospitals specializing in chronic and long-term illnesses. I have worked in nursing homes, I have spent years doing research for the World Health Organization (WHO), headed a geriatric department, and chaired and been part of many geriatric-related planning committees. Coming from this professional background, I feel knowledgeable enough to speak on the subject of quality of life during the later years. For a long time, I considered putting that knowledge into a book.

In the last few years I headed an agency providing home care. This allowed me to see the quality of daily life in different situations: that of an elderly person residing in a nursing home or in another institutional setting, and that of one residing in his or her own home. In this book I examine society's relationship to and with the elderly, as well as the organized cultural relationship with the aging population today. Evaluating the impact of today's family structure on the aged and their lifestyle, and how different this is from the familiar structure in the past, makes it clear how difficult it is to get older in these times.

One cannot discuss the subject of the aged without examining the economic implications on their lives. The policy makers at the state and the federal levels, as well as the city government level, at times are totally detached from the reality of everyday life of the elderly. How do we interrelate and consolidate all those aspects to produce a better, longer, and more fulfilling life for our elders, and how do we prepare ourselves for our own needs at the later years of our lives? Those are just a few of the topics that I will be discussing in this book.

Being in my late fifties myself gives me the ability to examine first-hand two totally different patterns of family practices and behavior:

the life that my parents' generation practiced, and the one that my generation is practicing. The fact that I was born into European culture also colors my experiences. Fifty years ago, one's mobility (in terms of residence) was limited due to economic, technical, and cultural restrictions. One was predestined to live close to family and, in most cases, die not far from the place he or she was born. Familiarity was the name of the game, and one did not venture out of his or her comfort zone too often.

Grandparents were an integral part of the family, in many ways, the foundation on which the family was built. The elders had direct input in everyday life, the customs, traditions, values, and religious practices.

The aging members of the family never needed to worry about where they would live in their later years or who would take care of them, when they would not be able to take care of themselves.

If we look back, just say, 100 or 200 years, the parents, as well as the grandparents always stayed in the family house, and one or more siblings were responsible for the care and well-being of the elders. There were no nursing homes or other formal arrangements to care for the elderly.

The elderly, who did not have relatives, or anyone to take responsibility for their well-being, were usually cared for by nuns or other religious or philanthropic organizations. One took care of his or her elders the same way one was sure that they would be taken care of by their children when they would reach old age.

After World War II, this changed significantly. Suddenly opportunities opened up to more than the rich. Suddenly the middle class and the lower middle class, and even the lower class, had in their grasp the possibility to move throughout the country for education and for economic opportunities. If, years ago, it was part of your daily ritual to sit down for dinner every evening with all the members of your family, suddenly, your child was at school 2000 miles and one time zone away from you. Holidays and their importance to traditional and cultural behavior slowly changed. Your child, exposed to professional opportunities in and around the area of his schooling, was more than likely not to return to his childhood neighborhood.

Most family communication now is through electronic channels, such as telephones, computers, etc.

These days, children are establishing their families far away from their parents, whom they might see no more than once a year. One might say that the considerably inexpensive airfares make it possible to travel to one's family with ease. Nonetheless, with the demands that our everyday lives put upon us, there is less and less time to do so. In my work, I see more and more elderly people who are on their own, trying not to burden their children with their problems, coping as best as they can.

In all fairness, many children do try to be an active component in their parents' lives, with more frequent visits; they are involved in their parents' decisions-making regarding health issues, financial issues, and other issues. Members of the extended family— i.e., cousins, nephews, and/or friends — sometimes fill the void children filled in the old times. But it is quite clear that the elderly are more and more on their own than ever before. And loneliness has become a given in their lives. In this book I shall discuss the options that our society offers to the elderly who are living on their own.

When we study the elderly and what ails them carefully, we see that the things that affect them most are: loneliness, isolation, hopelessness, helplessness, and lack of social contact and engagement in social and physical activities, bringing on boredom, and illness.

Many psychological studies show that the long-term effects of loneliness and isolation have a great impact on the health of the elderly: bringing on illness, prolonging recuperation from illness, complicating illness, and shortening life span. Not too many people will argue with the notion that one should not live alone and that loneliness and isolation are definitely not good for one's happiness and well being.

So what are the alternatives? The best one, of course, is for one to live at the later years of his or her life with or near family to provide an active support system. But if this not possible, what then? In this book you will find many different options and the pros and cons for each, to make it easier for you or your parent to evaluate the most suitable option for you.

There is the good old nursing home, but maybe it's not always so good. Let's look at this option more closely. I worked for many years in nursing homes, and I agree that at times it is the only viable option for the elderly. But by all means, try every other avenue available before choosing that one. In general, one can say that being institutionalized in a nursing home deters an individual from being just that, an individual. All decision-making is removed, and institutionalized routines totally take over every aspect of one's life. I will consider this option in depth later in this book.

In the last 20 years more and more retirement shared-living situations have become available to the elderly. Some of them are quite good. Most of them are built on beautiful grounds; some include luxury suites, tennis courts, golf, pools, and recreational programs. In some, one can find fancy dining arrangements, a nurse on the premises, a social worker, etc., and luxury amenities. The drawbacks of such a place are that it is geared to higher functioning individuals, and in most cases very independent individuals. Some places do not accommodate wheelchairs, or people with disabilities that require special provisions such as wide corridors, ramps, or elevators. There is sometimes internal pressure on the residents to be active and partake in all activities, far beyond what some can or want to do. And above all, these places tend to be highly priced and out of reach for most retired individuals.

Such shared-living situations also demand the individual to readjust to a new situation, new people, new routines, and a totally new environment. Although it is partially independent living, it is still very structured and regulated. If the person coming into such a situation is a shy individual, he or she is likely to be lonely and unengaged. You will find more on that option in the chapter dealing directly with shared-living facilities.

Shared households are also an option, although not in significant numbers. This option is appropriate for a highly functioning individual. It basically provides for two or more individuals sharing a residential household, for economic and social considerations.

This option is actually quite good. Expenses are cut in half or more. One is not alone, there is always someone there, and household chores are shared, making life much easier. Social interaction is built in.

But it also has some drawbacks.

Shared living has to be established with much care so several important components fit, with the understanding that if any one component is missing or unstable, it may cause the entire arrangement to fail. In the chapter dealing with the different residential options, this is explained in detail.

As said previously, the best of all possibilities is to remain at home. In the period when a person is not totally dependent on a caregiver, the elderly person may only require help with shopping, trips to the doctor's office, and some household chores. There are agencies that are available to step in for specified needs, i.e., Meals on Wheels, Access-a-Ride, etc. The problem with this set-up is that there is no coordination between sources of services, and the care is fragmented. This fragmentation may affect the care and be harmful to the senior, if, for example, one doctor does not know what medication other doctors are prescribing to him or her. With fragmented care, the well-being of the elderly, both mental and psychological, may be neglected.

In this situation, to provide a safe and nurturing environment for the elderly, a back-up support system should be in place. There should be a family member, a neighbor, or a friend to look in on the senior to make sure the needed help is provided. That designated person should be the one coordinating the different service providers, and making sure that all medical treatments are known among all specialists.

As we age, our decision-making becomes affected to some degree. That degree varies from person to person, and is directly related to age, health status, medication, and environment. Thus there is an essential need to have someone to help make important decisions, when one is unable to do so independently. But one must be careful to whom one designates to this role. Later in this book I will expand on the subject of power of attorney and health proxy, as well as the different trusts that are available and relate to the needs of the aged. The helpful ways to protect one's self are presented in the chapter dealing with legal considerations.

At some stage, most of the elderly will require greater care, as their ability to remain totally independent decreases. One of the choices is home care, which may be introduced as needed. An aide can be brought in to help with Activities of Daily Living (ADLs), as needed, for a few hours a day, only a few days a week, for example. Hours may be increased as the needs increase, eventually covering day and night care. If this is done through a qualified agency, it will come with a wide range of support systems.

This book was written with the premise to help you navigate through the landscape of health systems and guide you through the maze of options that are available to you. The idea is to make it easier for you to evaluate the best choices for your situation. I hope this book will guide you, and help you on this journey. For your convenience, the material has been arranged in chapters that concentrate on specific topics relating to aging, needs, and services. Throughout the book you will find cases of real clients of mine and their experiences.

I will try to answer the questions that we all ask, whether we are middle-aged children of aging parents, or just a population of people that are facing our own aging and preparing for the future. If anyone asked us how we see our lives in the later years, we would all say we'd like to be healthy, independent, socially and physically active, and not be a burden on our families. Well, let's explore the possibilities of maximizing our quality of life using what is available in the society we live in, regardless of the level of our independence or health status.

Chapter 1 –
The Aging of America – Are you ready?

Knowing the Elder

Before starting to evaluate the concept of retirement, we should begin with an understanding of the aging population in our society. This requires an open and honest discussion in which we need to look at what society has available for the elderly now and in the future.

If you consider that getting old is a natural progression of life, and we all age from the moment that we are born, it may be easier to think about the elder years, ours as well as those of the people around us.

We all understand that if we are not old at this time, we all will get there. Thus, all that I am considering in this book applies to us all, just at different times. For some, the time is now; for others it is still in the future. But we all have parents, neighbors, people that have a place in our hearts, people that may benefit, fully or partially, from the information in this book, right now.

If you currently provide care, either to a relative, or to someone unrelated, you too may benefit from the information in this book. For most, the knowledge that you are not alone in this situation helps a great deal. But we should understand that the issues dealing with old age, life quality of the elderly, and care relate to the old and the young and those in between. Same issues touch the giver, some touch the receiver, and some issues touch both. And for the care to be successful and beneficial to both parties, it requires good channels of communication.

When we initiate communication with the elderly, we need to be sensitive in preserving their dignity. I am sure that as we age, we lose some of the confidence that we had in the younger years. Many of us

1

have difficulties accepting the fact that we are dependent on others. There may be times that important decisions are made for us, and some people treat us as if we are imbeciles at worst, or children at best. I cannot stress strongly enough how important it is to preserve the dignity of the elderly and to treat them with respect.

The following are some guidelines for respecting the elderly, and preserving their dignity:

1. When speaking to the elderly, make sure that you are at the same eye level and you do not look down at them. This brings the sense of equality to both of you.

2. When you sit across from the elderly, make sure that there is a respectable distance between you. A proper amount of space will show respect, while too much space projects coldness and detachment.

3. Speak clearly and directly, and speak loudly if you know he or she has a hearing deficiency.

4. Invite the elder to have input in decision-making that will affect his or her life. Invite them to make choices. This way they will not have the sense that they are losing control of their situation, and that things are being decided for them.

5. Make sure that they are aware that you respect their opinions, preferences, and possessions.

6. Encourage them to have input in their own care. For as long as they are able to do some of the tasks in their home, or care for their own personal needs, let them do it for themselves.

7. Always *offer* to help, rather than insist on helping them. Verbalize what you are about to do, so they do not perceive a sudden movement as a threat.

8. If you control their finances, make sure that they have some money in their wallet; this makes them retain some sense of adulthood. Do not question them as to what they did with the money in their wallet as this will make them feel like a child, needing to account for every dollar.

Getting older is a family affair. And we should be attuned to the fact that the elderly want to remain independent, in their home, and be the least possible burden to their family.

We should sit down with our elders and discuss their expectations for their later years. This discussion should take place on the personal level, with one's family.

The key question of the day is whether society at large is ready to cope with the growing number of aging members in its midst. Beyond providing elevators at subway stations or kneeling buses, the health care system has to provide services that are geriatric in nature and available in the numbers appropriate for an increasingly aging population. And if society is not ready, there is very precious little time to get ready.

So the evaluation of the topic of aging should take place on two levels, one of which that relates to the society at large with its communal issues and subjects that affect large segments of population. The other relates to the individual dealing with her or his plans for the senior years, or the issues and plans related to elderly parents or an aging spouse.

Let's begin with the need to review the topic on an individual level. I remember that as a young woman, aging seemed like such a strange thing. When I was 20, 40 looked so old. Yet, when I reached the age of 40, it seemed so young to me. Now that I am reaching the end of my fifties, and the sixties are just around the corner, the fifties seem quite young. On the occasions that I do think of the process of aging, I can't ignore the fact that my seventies and even the eighties are not that far off.

We all know that one day we will be senior citizens, but somehow, it is easier to see the person next to us aging, without relating this to ourselves. How many times have you met someone that you did not see for a long time, and thought, "Oh, my God, he has aged so much." I am sure there are people saying that about me, but when I look in the mirror, I do not see myself as almost 60. The old age seems to be pushed away; it's always on the horizon, but we never really reach it in our minds.

So when do we begin to feel like "seniors," "elders," or plain "old?" Never, in my opinion. We never really feel old, unless one is ill. Sickness can make one feel quite old, and quickly. But our society does provide us with set guidelines as to when we are considered seniors. It is the built-in retirement age; it is the time that we qualify for Social Security or Medicare. That's the time that the label begins to stick, even though in our minds we are still thinking of ourselves as middle-aged or young.

Society tells us that at 65 years for women, or 67 years for men, we are seniors. For most of us it is far too early to consider ourselves seniors. But it is nonetheless a good time to review our life in the context of what our needs may be in the future, not only health-wise, but also in the social and everyday-life aspects.

Most of us will quickly say that we do not feel old, and the time ahead of us seems vast, that there is no need to be pressured with all the legalities, planning, and decision-making. If there is any way that I can convince you, please do take the time to consider your future, as well as that of your parents. The future is here, and now is the time to start to evaluate how best to plan and prepare.

Even the healthiest of us at some point slow down. Our bodies start to show signs of aging, reflexes are not as sharp as they were, and our reaction time begins to slow down. Joints that carried us through our youth and middle age start to show the wear and tear. You may still feel quite youthful inside your head, but your body tells you differently. That is in all probability the first time in your life that the word "senior" is used in relation to you.

Not all of us retire as soon as we hit the age of 65. Some of us are quite happy to continue working and maintaining a productive life well into our seventies. There are others who cannot stop working because of financial pressures and the need to make ends meet. Some of us were never able to save for the later years of our lives, and some just thought that the later years would somehow be paid for by the government, or maybe by our kids, or maybe by hitting the lottery.

Other than Social Security, which may or may not still be around for the next generation, the workers who have some pension set up for them for future years are in the minority. Most of us do not have pensions. I do not think you need to be reminded how some large corporations, which previously had pensions for their workers, have squandered it, leaving their workers with no pension upon retirement. So the insecurity is still there, even if you are the lucky one working for a company that does provide a pension to its workers.

So a person aging today has to think very carefully about how he or she will invest their savings to last them throughout their retirement years. If your parents do not have any assets, or any kind of savings, they will be able to qualify for Medicaid, a government program that will provide for their home care assistance or nursing home, if they should need it. You will find more information in the chapter on Medicaid.

It is not always easy to have conversations on the sensitive subjects of financial, legal, and medical issues. Your parents may not be receptive to you asking them questions regarding their finances, where they keep legal papers, or whether all their insurance policies are up to date. But this conversation needs to take place for their own protection.

Often, when a parent or spouse needs help, the family comes together, each pulling an equal share in responsibilities and care. But in this imperfect world, where siblings live all over the United States, it is hard to provide the care for your parent or elder with equal shares of commitment. If there had been problems among the siblings over the years and relations were strained, it is likely that this will be reflected in the sharing of the care of their parent. The care receiver will most likely sense it and be distraught over it. This type of situation should best be avoided if possible.

If one of the siblings lives far away and is therefore not able to provide his or her share of help, he or she can pay for the care to be provided by an aide, thus making it more equal in sharing the load. But in many cases the sharing of care can bring with it many unhappy feelings. It is essential that open discussions be held from the start, and individual responsibilities determined in advance. It may also be advisable to put the final agreement in writing, so that there are no misunderstandings.

The family, the elderly, as well as the caregiver, need to understand the differences between physical illness and the mental implication of illness on the older person. Although most illnesses do not differentiate between the older and younger patient, how they affect them may be quite different.

Most diseases strike the elderly more often than young people. How diseases manifest themselves, and what symptoms they present, can be quite different in people depending on their age. An underactive or overactive thyroid, for example, can produce symptoms of confusion in the elderly, but not in the young person with the same illness. It is very important that proper diagnosis be made, and that the elderly person is not misdiagnosed with dementia. This is so important because the patient needs to be treated for the underlying disease.

As the medical field is achieving a great deal of advances in the diagnosing and treatment of illness, the diseases that outright killed many not many years ago have become mostly chronic illnesses. We live longer, even with those diseases; though treating them requires a coordinated effort with doctors' visits and a routine of medication and follow up, not to mention the cost of treatment for these diseases.

Some of the illnesses striking the elderly tend to be debilitating, requiring much assistance from either the family or an aide. But the level of assistance varies, depending on the stage of the disease, and may be stepped up as the need increases. Even so, some help may be needed from the start. So it is important to be somewhat prepared before a crisis presents itself.

Many of us are ill-prepared to deal with illnesses that are chronic, from which we will not get better. If we or someone we love is ill, the stress that we go through can get the best of us. One of the ways to reduce stress is to familiarize ourselves with the illness, as well as with the treatment for it. Seek out information from the doctor who is treating you or your loved one, from the Internet, and from published material on the subject. As hard as it may be, it is wise to be prepared and to know what is to be expected with the progression of the disease.

If the illness requires hospitalization, the hospitals will provide the care the patient needs. The hospital offers health care providers and social workers to guide you and prepare you for the time you or your loved one is discharged.

At the time of discharge you should be prepared to deal with whatever needs you may encounter upon returning home. If assistance is needed with daily care, that should be prearranged prior to discharge. Besides being informed as to the physical and medical needs that the patient will require upon returning home, his or her psychological needs should also be provided for, if needed.

When you care for your loved one, you need to take into account the toll this care will take on you. The time you spend with your parent is time taken away from yourself and from your family. Your children or your spouse may feel short-changed by your absence from them. The care you give to your parent may stress you, may render you continuously tired, physically and emotionally. You should not downplay it.

While providing care for others, you should not forget yourself.

If at all possible, encourage your family to help you with the care. Their involvement need not be very taxing on them. They can simply visit, read to the senior, do their nails, share some news events, etc.

The help of your children and spouse with your parent or elderly relative will not only be actual help to you, but also will make them more understanding and sensitive to the needs of those they are helping. In my experience, you tend to feel better about yourself and the world around you when you connect with the needs of others.

If care is provided by you and you alone, and there is no support or understanding from those around you, eventually you may start feeling resentment and stress, feelings that may impact your daily life. To prevent that, you must have open channels of communication and encourage others, relatives and friends, to help out.

Discussions among siblings, friends, and relatives are essential for good understanding and venting, but they should not take place in front of the parent or elder that is in need of the care you are providing. The parent or elder should not feel that he or she is a burden to you. In my experience, personal and professional, most families that do not place blame on anyone, measure how much each person helped out, will come to a mutual understanding as to the task at hand.

Sharing equally is the best of solutions. But this may not always be possible. As adults, we should understand that the facts of life may not always allow us to share equally in the care of our loved one.

Geography - the distance of where we live in relation to our parents - our individual family situation, and responsibilities, including having our own young children, may affect our ability to provide substantive care for our parent. But if the understanding is there, all involved will feel much better, and less stressed.

We may also feel unappreciated by our parent whom we care for. If our parent did not openly show appreciation for things that we did for them in the past, it is a given that they will not show much appreciation for what we do for them now. We should not expect them to change at their old age. Some of them will not show appreciation because they have a hard time admitting that they are needy.

If your parent or dear one behaves much differently from the way he or she behaved in the past, this may be due to an illness. This should be brought to the attention of the family doctor so it can be addressed.

If you feel frustrated, it would be advisable to vent, to have a support system, or a shoulder to lean on. Carrying emotional stress will impact you negatively and affect your everyday life and health.

If the care you provide for a parent or a loved one affects your employment or your earnings, you should know that under the Family and Medical Leave Act (1993), you may take 12 weeks of leave, without worrying that you will lose your position at your place of employment. Some estimates peg the free care provided by family members or friends, at over $200 billion a year.

If you have to provide care to your parent from afar, you should resist the first inclination to relocate your parent to be near you. It may not always be the best move for them. Allow time to think things over, and to consider other options.

Evaluate your parent's situation. Use professional help when needed and available, to assess the situation. Speak to your parent's doctor regarding medical status and care needed on a daily basis. You can make arrangements for a home health aide, set in motion care providers and special programs, such as Access-a-Ride, Meals on Wheels, etc., so their daily needs are provided. That will help give you time to make the decisions without pressure.

Make sure to establish a support system around your parent. You may use friends, siblings, distant relatives, anybody that can be of help. The help does not have to be extensive; it can be a visit here and there, a call to check on them. Be available if an emergency occurs. During snow storms and hurricanes make sure that they are okay, and have basic supplies in their home (See the list of items in the chapter that deals with planning for emergencies).

Explain to relatives, neighbors, and friends that when they visit your parent they should be alert to signs of trouble. They should notify you if they notice upon visiting your parent that the house or apartment is neglected, that your parent looks dirty and unkempt, that there are foul odors in the house, or your parent seems to have lost a significant amount of weight. These visitors provide extra sets of eyes. And if you are notified, you have to act upon this information, because it may signal serious problems.

If you do not have any relatives near your parents or any neighbors willing to help, you may want to notify the post office that services your parent's street to keep an eye open for any signs of trouble. If mail is not picked up for a day or two, if lights are on throughout the day, if shutters are closed for a day or two, they should notify the police so they can check.

You may want to speak to the police precinct that covers your parent's neighborhood to be aware that your parent lives alone, and ask them to pass by the home from time to time to check on your parent. Most police and sheriff departments will check on the elderly, and make sure that they are all right in times of excessive heat, snowstorms, and hurricanes.

Some of the utility companies, such as telephone, electric and gas companies have established programs such as Elder Watch. Those programs are designed to be sensitive to signs that something may be wrong. You can call your local utility company and ask if they have such a program, and what you need to do to be part of it.

If you and your siblings live far away from your parent, and even from each other, and your parent is reaching a stage in which he or she cannot live alone, yet financially you would like to push back the option of paid care or moving your parent to a care facility, you may consider sharing daily care expenses with your sibling. Your parent may stay with you perhaps for 6 months and then be moved to your sibling for 6 months. This arrangement may work for a while, if each of you has a home that can accommodate an elderly person who may also have some physical problems. This option will require full support of all the members of your family because it will affect them all.

If your home or your sibling's home have many stairs, it may be difficult for the elderly to use them. If there is no additional room for your dear one, it may be fine for them to stay in the living room for a few days, but it will be very inconvenient for them, as well as for you and your family, to maintain this arrangement long-term.

It may be more convenient for all involved to rotate the stay with your parent. For example, you may agree that you will stay a few weeks with your parent, in his or her house, and then your sibling, a child of yours or theirs, or a relative, will stay with them for the next few weeks.

You and your siblings must meet as often as needed to discuss the care of your parent. If there is an acute change in your parent's health and the level of care needs to be changed, the situation needs to be reassessed. If there is a change of mental status, such as increased confusion, or greater memory loss, or if there are noticeable behavioral changes, they need to be discussed with all the involved parties.

Behavioral changes are at times hard to define. Some elderly are very good at masking mental changes, such as confusion (see the chapter on dementia), and lapses in memory. If you notice aggressive behavior or verbal or physical abusiveness - against you or others, or even against pets, plants, or furniture, this may be a sign that intervention is needed. This should be discussed among members of the family, and followed through with appropriate medical care.

One can use family gatherings and holiday get-togethers to have discussions regarding the needs of a parent. Whenever possible, include your parent in the discussion of their care, and let them express themselves as to how they see the care or what they would like. But disagreements among siblings should not be voiced in the presence of the parent, if she or he is the subject of the disagreements.

You should use the occasions that you meet with your siblings to discuss issues related to your parents. All legal papers should be reviewed by all of you. All siblings should be aware of a will, health proxy, insurance policies, and any other instructions that your parent put in place. If there are any special instructions regarding medical decisions that your parents would like you to carry out on their behalf, all of the siblings should be made aware of them. All siblings should also be made aware of where all legal papers are kept.

Having everyone on the same page will help to avoid stress and tensions among members of the family if/when emergencies arrive. If there are insurance policies in place, make sure there are no duplications, for example, two policies that essentially cover the same thing, insurance policies being paid for a spouse who died already, or insurance for a car that they no longer have. Review all legal papers as well as bank accounts. Check if checks have been written out to unknown persons, or for receipts for shopping that they did not do. In this book, you will find some examples of scams perpetuated against the elderly, and it will alert you to the need to protect your parent and yourself.

Case # 1

A few years back my home health care agency took care of a nice elderly gentleman, Mr. H., who lived on his own until his mid 80's, and kept a very organized, clean house. He was social and easily engaged in conversation. For a long time he had fooled the people around him, making a good job of hiding his confusion and forgetfulness.

Prior to Mr. H. becoming our patient, I had spoken with him on two occasions. We had short and simple conversations, in which I detected some slight confusion, though its severity didn't dawn on me until later. At the first meeting I had given him my business card.

A few weeks later, I received a call from a local hospital, notifying me that Mr. H. was found drunk, with a broken hand, in the middle of the night. He was brought in to the emergency room by a police officer. He was disoriented and unable to give any personal information. In his wallet, the emergency room staff found my business card, so they called me.

Mr. H. was discharged to our agency's care. We had him evaluated mentally and medically. Physically, other than the broken hand, he was okay. Mentally was another matter. He was diagnosed with Alzheimer's disease. He had a drinking problem. And he had no family to look after him. So we established a care system, providing him with a home care aide for eight hours a day, seven days a week. He was fighting us on that, refusing to see the need for someone to do things for him, such as cleaning and shopping, and personal care.

In a very short time, we discovered that Mr. H. had been taking out large sums of money from his bank account, and spending it in the local bar, paying for drinks for all of the bar's patrons. He was basically buying friendship. As he was going there daily, giving out his money, even his bank officer noticed that thousands of dollars were being withdrawn.

I tried to talk to him, but he did not remember taking money from the bank, or paying for all those "buddies" of his. Yet, when evening came, he would go out, as if on automatic pilot, to the nearest bar. Then the aide started to notice that Mr. H. was receiving suspicious phone calls with demands of all sorts of payment. He was confused and apologetic, and always promised to pay whatever it was the callers said he owed them.

Mr. H's care was extended to 24 hours a day, after an episode in which he left his house, and in confusion was unable to find his way back. He was found by the police wandering around barefoot, and without a coat, during a cold winter night. After that episode, we understood that he could not be left alone for any part of the day or night. Having an aide in his home day and night, we discovered other scams. There was a woman who showed up weekly, claiming to be his wife; this was proven not to be true. She would demand money from him, and he would give it to her. His "buddies" from the bar, had a game going; call Mr. H. and tell him that he owes them $500 or $700 for an x-ray, or for work on a car that he did not have. He always paid them.

At this time we found a cousin, one that was willing to take some interest in Mr. H.'s affairs and establish some measure of protection for him. We screened the calls that demanded money. We notified the Protective Services every time we had information on a person trying to scam Mr. H.

In place of a bar visit, we began a daily routine of taking him to the local donut store. He was very happy to have a cup of coffee and a donut, for which he paid himself, and enjoyed the excursion very much. His social interaction needs were satisfied by having a social and caring aide, and participating in social activities in the neighborhood senior citizen center.

Whatever money was left in Mr. H.'s bank accounts covered his home care as well as his living expenses. When his assets were depleted, we processed him for Medicaid. He stayed in his home until the last week of his life. His Alzheimer's progressed, robbing him of his personality, of his world, and all that he knew in it. But he was sweet and gentle until he died. Whenever I visited him and tried to engage him in any kind of communication, he would smile, look at me, or rather, through me, not knowing who I was, or even who he was.

Now, many years later, whenever I think about Mr. H., I cannot help but think of all the people who are alone and have no one to stand up for them and protect them and their money.

More protective regulation need to be put in place for banks to look out for signs of improper withdrawal of funds. Neighbors should look out for the elderly in their midst. And family should be connected, and protective, and be there for them.

I will continually stress how much we have to be on guard and watch out for signs of trouble of an elderly person being a victim of neglect. Whether physical or mental abuse, steps should be taken to protect the elderly. We have to look carefully at the people around us, because we may be the only eyes that are looking out for them at a given time.

No personal requests from people you know little of, or not at all, should be honored. In my agency, we had home health aides and personal assistants sign an agreement, protecting the patient, to whose home we sent them. In this agreement, on which they were also in-serviced, they were asked not to encourage financial discussions, not to ask the patient about their finances, not to ask them for loans, however small, and not to share with the patient their personal problems or financial difficulties. The patient was encouraged as well not to pay, or reward in any other manner, the worker for his or her good work. They were advised that workers are well paid by their agencies and the only gifts one should give is optional for the worker's birthday. And such a gift should be a token present, so no future expectations are promoted.

Case # 2

Ms. G. was referred to my agency by her family member. She was 97 years old at the time, and up to that time living on her own, in an apartment that she lived in for 44 years. She was fully alert and her level of mental sharpness would put many young people to shame.

Ms. G. was financially very well off and although she did not have children of her own, and did not hesitate to tell you her opinion on the marital institution, she did have an extended family of nephews and nieces. She was nobody's fool, and informed me at our first meeting that her family members had shown up in the later years of her life. Finding out her net worth, they suddenly displayed love for their aunt.

One night, Ms. G. fell in her apartment and broke her hip, going from hospital to rehabilitation. With her mobility permanently decreased, her nephew transferred her to an assisted living facility. He called me to ask if we could provide an aide for his aunt to help with basic needs. He was very proud of himself that he succeeded to get her into a facility that cost her $5,500 a month. This did not include meals. And she was asked not to come down to the dining room; wheelchairs did not look too good. We safe-proofed her apartment and brought her back home. From that point on, Ms. G. had 24 hour care for 7 days a week.

We established a routine that Ms. G. liked. Her social life continued and she attended parties, given by different organizations, and senior citizen centers. She maintained involvement with family and friends. Her aides bathed her, kept her house clean, took her to her doctor's appointments, and cooked her meals. Many times she said "this is what I worked for all my life, to live out my years in the comfort of my home, with the help I need. I love living in my home with the things I love and hold dear". Ms. G. lived to a ripe old age of 103.

The Target Population

In the year 2030, twenty percent of the total population in this country will be 65 years and older. Most will be retired by then due to the somewhat shrinking labor market (automatization and outsourcing being the main causes). Improved health services and availability of programs that promote better knowledge of maintaining good health add years to the life of the aging population.

The projected numbers for baby boomers are that, within 10 years of when they join the senior Americans, there will be some 77 million people 55 and older. The first of the baby boomers are beginning to enter the golden age, joining the ranks of the already high numbers of seniors. As of today, 1 million people aged 65 years and older live in New York State.

The following statistics came from the U.S Census Bureau, U.S. Department of Health and Human Services, and American Association of Home Services for the Aging:

Americans age 65 and older in 2007:   37,462,000
Americans age 65 and older projected in 2020:   54,632,000
Americans in need of long-term care in 2007:   9,000,000
Americans in need of long-term care projected in 2020: 12,000,000

Although old age is slow to develop, and does so mostly unnoticed, one day, you suddenly find that it is upon you. Most of us do not notice that we are aging until we have already aged. The first sign that we have reached that point is when we receive the Social Security information kit. But the baby-boomer generations that are coming up are for the most part a different breed.

Baby boomers make up a highly educated group, as a whole. They are physically much more fit than the generations before them. Many of them planned for their retirement better, and their investments in general are directed for their later years. This is of course a generalization, and there are many that fall out of this projection.

The baby boomers have also been much more engaged in social and political issues. The economic environment in the United States allowed them to be a much more vocal population in society. I am sure that they will be actively pressuring their elected officials to develop programs that are geared towards improving their lives. The increasing number of people over 50 carries great power, and that can be translated into almost unlimited benefits for that specific population. We are smartening up to it. It is just a matter of time.

Health services in America today are better than they were for previous generations. But they are still not available to everybody, and even for those who have access, there is varying levels of care. With health insurance being in mostly the private sector, the cost varies so greatly that it makes no sense to even compare it. It varies from state to state, from one insurance company to another. The benefits offered change randomly and the changes are not based on any rationale at all, except the financial gains from which the insurance companies are benefiting. This is the haphazard system that provides the health services for the American people.

So who are the baby boomers that are moving out of middle age into the senior citizen realm? Statistically they are more educated, computer savvy, able to access greater pools of knowledge, and thus, practice better personal health. They are better at following good nutritional habits, and understand what they need to do to maintain good health.

With all that said, it is still a roll of the dice whether one will develop a debilitating disease. Environmental and genetic causes still inflict those diseases and their complications upon us. As longevity increases, society as a whole has to be aware of the implications of such longevity. People living longer with debilitating illness require more specialized care and more costly care. Although we as Americans have not reached a point where we equally provide health insurance to all our citizens, we will be the ones that have to foot the bill for the care of our seniors.

Medicare and Medicaid are the programs now providing coverage for the elderly and others who are unable to afford medical care. These services have been stretched by the growing number of seniors in need, when at the same time the federal government has been cutting the funds.

Health cost has become so ridiculously high and does not provide satisfactory dollar-for-dollar return in services to the public. The health industry is powerful, with one of the most powerful lobbies, that gives it a great pull in Washington, thus influencing the laws and regulations that govern our benefits. And the government doesn't always seem to look out for the good of its people. We should remember that at election time. A good example for that is the refusal to allow Medicare to negotiate the prices of medications for Medicare Part D.

If America is to fulfill its obligations to its seniors, it needs to begin with offering them a system where their medical and physical needs are met. But unfortunately, not only the elderly are insufficiently insured, but some 45 million Americans of all ages are not insured at all. In this book, I would like to show some ways to ensure that you, your parent, friend, or relative finds a venue to find coverage for his or her health needs.

It may feel at times that you are in a situation no one else understands, or has ever experienced, but you are not alone. There are millions of elderly, millions of their kids, middle aged people that deal with their elderly parents, and their own aging. When I started to compile material for this book, my intended target population was seniors, but very quickly I realized that the subject touches us all. We all have parents, grandparents, aging relatives, and neighbors; we should educate ourselves as to the options available for all of us.

We all want to do well for our parents, elderly, the ill, and the disabled. But our society, as rich as it is, has poorly prepared us for the task. Most of us do not know where to reach out for help and guidance. Things are not arranged to make it easy for us. It is a constant voyage of discovery.

As we travel on this voyage, we learn about ourselves, our parents, the elderly, and society in general, and our relationships to everyone else. It relates not only to care-giving, but also to care-receiving. How we relate to the elderly will color our own aging, and the life we will lead at our old age. Concentrating on ours and others' dignity, social connection, sense of place, and family commitments, will allow us to grow old happier. I read the following statement years ago, and it stuck with me.

"GROWING OLD IS MANDATORY, GROWING UP IS OPTIONAL."

- Chili Davis

One can look at the task of caring for one's parent as repayment for all they gave us. Your parents gave you life; they nurtured you when you were a child. Caring for one's parent can bring openness that you may not have had throughout your life and up to that point. It is the optimal gift you can give to a human being, relative or not, by caring for them in the period in their life when they need it most.

Our culture places high value on self reliance. We do not want to acknowledge weakness and neediness. That is true for us as well as for our elders. But as we age, we all need help, some of us more than others.

Society should be reeducated as to how we should deal with our elders, in caring for them in a respectful way. We should include them in our society fully. As long as they are able mentally and physically, they should be made to feel that they are important, productive, and adding to society. And they are. They bring with them knowledge and a wealth of experiences. Even if physically they may not be able to actively help others, they can bring to the table years and years of what they know, what they have done in their lives, and what lessons they may have learned.

But now as the older population is growing, we need to make major changes in our society, in the way we view old age, relate to it, and deal with it. While we build a society that is sensitive to the problems of the elderly, and make their elder years better, so will our life become better, when we get older. We, the members of our society, regardless of our age, need to take greater responsibility for one another, the way early societies did.

In 2005, 80 percent of elder care was given by a family member, or someone close to the care receiver in the United States. The estimated value of unpaid work (annually) is as high as $257 billion by some sources. One needs not to be an economist to understand the implications of those numbers on the economy.

Women shoulder the responsibility for care more often then men. The AARP's National Alliance for Care Giving found that a typical care giver is a woman, 46 years old, married, working outside of her home, and earning $35,000.

One of the issues that our society has to come to grips with is the need to have open conversation with our elders. We should deal with issues of aging and disability. In many cases the elderly are resistant to such conversation. It scares them. Nonetheless, the subject should be broached delicately and at the tempo that is dictated by the elderly.

The questions to be asked are:

1. How is their health status at the time of conversation? What is the prognosis?

2. Is the home a viable place for them to live? Is the home safe for them?

3. What adjustments need to be made? Should a new arrangement be made?

4. Do they need assistance with routine activities of daily living?

5. What is their financial situation?

6. To whom should you delegate the responsibility of making health-related decisions? Where should documents such as the will, insurance policies, burial directives, and banking statements be stored?

7. Do they have long-term insurance? Is it adequate?

8. End of life wishes?

9. Planning for sources of care, if relatives have to direct them long distance.

Most of us are so busy with our lives, that we hardly notice the aging process of our parents, and one day, due to some event, an accident or an illness, we suddenly realize that our parents have aged, and here the strong and independent people we relied on, are helpless and needy. And now we are the ones that have to help them, and look after them. As mentioned before, they are not always willing to let us step in.

But our parents and elderly in general, do need us. And more than that, they cannot go it alone anymore. Just as our parents are unable to pinpoint the moment that the change occurs, so are we often oblivious to the fact that our parents are now unable to care for themselves.

When do we step in, and how do we know it is time?

Here are some signs that should trigger warnings:

1. Personal care: Your parent, who always was neat, suddenly is wearing stained clothing, missing buttons, has body odor, is uncombed, and/or is neglecting his or her personal hygiene.

2. Home care: Is the household dirty? Are bills unpaid? Is there garbage around the house and spoiled food in the refrigerator? Are the carpets stained? Are the bed sheets soiled? Are your parents reluctant to accept outside help?

3. Food: Is there a decrease in appetite? Is the refrigerator empty or full of uneaten food? Are there notable signs of weight loss? Check for denture problems, and if applicable, chewing problems.

4. Memory loss: Do they call you at work, or in the middle of the night? Do they call a few times during the day not remembering that they already called, or do they repeat whatever it is that they wanted to tell you?

5. Communication: Does your parent have difficulties following directions? Do they frequently search for the right word during conversations, or get confused by the phone or remote control?

6. Mobility: Does your parent have difficulties going up and down stairs? Are they able to get up from a soft chair by themselves? Can they get out of a car from a sitting position, unassisted?

7. Depression: Do they present a loss of interest in life? If your parents were readers, television watchers, or sport lovers, and show noticeable loss of interest in those things, it should be a warning sign. Have they lost interest in food? Have they stopped being social, though they were social before? Are they becoming angry and moody for no apparent reason? (It could be due to mental changes, or physical changes, as well as to incorrect usage of medication.)

8. Medication: Do you find in your parent's medicine cabinet medication with expired dates, maybe partially used? Are bottles too full and not used timely and as directed? Do they finish their medication too soon, by taking too much? Are they purchasing their medications in different pharmacies? Do they have too many over-the-counter medications, such as aspirin, cough syrup, and antacids?

9. Finances: Have you noticed that your parents paid a bill twice? Or did not pay a bill that was due? Have they misplaced checks? Are you noticing a great deal of unopened mail, or notices from collection agencies?

10. Driving: Are you noticing an increase in traffic violations, minor accidents, scratches, or dents that your parents cannot explain? Do they ever get lost while driving to familiar places? Do you need to call your parents to check that they arrived home all right? Are you uncomfortable being in your parents' car, while they are driving?

If we look around our own immediate environment, such as our place of work, our neighborhood, or our social circle, we hear of many parents, neighbors, or relatives that are struggling with illness and mental deficiencies. My mother always said "The one thing I fear at my old age is losing my mental capacity to judge what is right and what is wrong." Losing one's ability to think, decide, recognize, and remember must be worse than having any other illness.

How do we recognize the slow deterioration of our parents' mental ability? In the chapter pertaining to dementia, I will provide you with an overview of the loss of mental abilities. The information will help you to familiarize yourself with different dementia conditions and how they manifest themselves. If the signs of dementia present themselves in your dear one, you will need to seek professional help.

Baby Boomers

In the coming years, the baby boomer generation will enter the long-term care and special health care needs market in unprecedented numbers. Born in the years between 1946 and 1964, the so-called baby boomers have had a profound effect on public policy at every stage of their lives thus far. As the years go on and the baby boomer generation requires nursing home services more and more, we as a society will be faced with the challenge of redefining long-term care. We need to recognize the needs of this generation, or it will break the backbone of the health care system.

In just a few years we will have a population of 78 million people over the age of 60. All of them will require, sooner or later, some degree of health care services. Our society has to be ready for it. This requires a great deal of preparation.

The complicating factor in this situation is the fact that the United States does not have a universal health system. Unlike poorer nations, that do provide universal health systems, we have a health system that is fractioned and uneven, with millions falling in the cracks with no health coverage at all. Many more millions of Americans that do have insurance and think they are covered in a time of need, are either only partially covered, or not covered at all for specific needs.

We do not have health coverage for every child or adult in this country, much less coverage for all of our elders. Both ends of the spectrum of our population are the neediest, yet they are not covered in a satisfactory way.

As of today, we do not have enough medical facilities, laboratories, doctors, nurses, gerontologists and geriatric staff to accommodate the numbers that will flow in to the 60-years-and-over population. I am not an economist and therefore cannot paint a precise picture of what we will face economically when the full brunt of the pressure of cost materializes as more baby boomers become 60 and over. But it is sure to provide a tremendous blow to the general economy.

There is also the likelihood that the aging boomers' generation will force society to rethink the way it sees old age and the way it provides for the elderly.

During the early childhood years of the baby boomers' generation, a great deal of developments occurred. Diseases such as diphtheria, small pox and polio, which once killed and crippled children, were almost totally eradicated, or rendered almost harmless. Vaccinations for measles, chicken pox, rubella, and mumps became standard, and are routinely given to children in this country today.

The baby boomers have grown up in a society that has seen numerous medical advancements, and has practiced better habits. The development of the television media brought into American homes knowledge of better nutrition, although one can say that it also brought in to the homes the fast food mentality, which has had a negative effect on eating habits.

There are clear indications that the baby boomers are much healthier and much more active than the previous generation, participating in society in more productive and fulfilling ways. The development of better diagnostic tools, better medications and treatments, as well as genetic tools to either prevent debilitating diseases or help identify and treat them successfully, are all helping the boomers live longer and in better health.

Even so, they still have to deal with the health system if they or their spouses become chronically or terminally ill. Statistically, the cases are there, and they too have to deal with issues of care, either at home or in a different setting.

With such a large influx of seniors into the health system, the whole system will have to change the way it provides services. Currently, the health system is built mostly on providing acute care. You get sick, we try to cure you, or maintain you as best as the system is able. But in fact, most of the ill are chronically ill, with illness such as diabetes, high blood pressure, and heart disease. Although our population is getting older, the system is not preparing itself to deal with the oncoming problems, and the growing numbers of seniors in need of care.

We have to establish facilities that are representative of the needs of the baby boomers. We also need to force the long-term care services to become consumer friendly and consumer-oriented in order to make this a service-driven industry. This population, as stated before, is better educated, healthier, and better tuned to their physical needs, than any generation before them. They are computer-literate for the most part, and can seek out the information needed to plan, reach, and educate themselves for health needs. The government-related agencies, the gerontologists, the doctors, nurses, social workers, health professionals of all kinds, should make sure that such information is available to the boomer generation - to prepare them as best as possible to face their needs as they reach their senior years.

With the rapid increase in the demands for services for the aging population, we will need to make available to them more medical services, such as equipment for testing, laboratories, doctors, nurses, and pharmaceuticals. We also need to make sure that all the different residential options are available for them. It is true that the market has its ways to fulfill the need when the need presents itself, but many elderly people will not have the ability to pay for the options the market will offer them.

The government should start planning now for the future of our seniors. If you are active politically, you may want to write to your congressman and your senator to encourage them to work for the change in the general perception that makes us concentrate only on the young, while neglecting the old.

Case # 3

In my building, in which I have been living for the last 22 years, there are a great number of elderly people. Most of them have been living in this building since it was built, yet very few are friendly with one another, or are known to the newer tenants.

Over the years I have tried to become friends with some of them. I succeeded with a few, but in general they keep to themselves. Because of my background, I tried to break through their isolation. Younger people in the building tend to be engrossed in their own lives, and are unaware of their elderly neighbors. We all know how demanding every-day life is; we leave our homes in the morning, and do not return until late in the evening. Thus, we rarely know what is happening to our next-door neighbors.

Every few months an ambulance would stop in front of our building, responding to a call from an elderly person reaching out for help. I would ask the doorman what happened, and he would say, "oh, the lady from 5C...or the gentleman from 11H..." I have to admit that, most times, I did not know who the person was.

Two years ago, someone living on an upper floor called the doorman to report that there was a foul odor in the hallway. After some checking we realized that an elderly lady living alone in one of the apartments had not been seen for at least a few days, maybe more. Nobody could actually pinpoint when she was last seen.

The police were called, and upon breaking the door down, the elderly lady was found after she had been dead for some time. She was found on the floor, close to the door, in all likelihood trying to get out, maybe in an effort to reach out for help.

I realized, after that day, that there are too many lonely people, and there are too few safety nets out there for them. There are elderly people whose mental and physical health decline slowly, and at times no one is there to notice it. Some of them don't eat properly or maintain good health. In many cases, the society around them is too late to notice and step in to set things right, to help the elderly live out their lives as well as possible.

So, I have made it a point to introduce myself to as many elderly neighbors as possible. Some of them were quite suspicious of me, and I am sure that they were convinced I had some kind of ulterior motive. I gave them my personal number so they can call me any time they need help. I also told them which apartment was mine so they could ring the bell, if they needed to.

And they did ring the bell or call me—not all, but some. For some I arranged Access-a-Ride, so they had no difficulties getting to the doctor. I picked up stamps for some, or other items, to make their life a little easier.

It is not that I want to tell you how wonderful I am in helping the aged, it is that we all need to be educated in the importance of looking out for the elderly that are among us. I know that we would all be quite happy to know that our parents' neighbors are looking out for them if they are living far from us.

In a multi-dwelling building, one person who should definitely be alert to its elderly residents is the doorman or a superintendent. They should be instructed on how to notice the worrisome signs, such as confusion, increased forgetfulness, if the elderly resident is not seen a day or two, and has not informed anybody that he or she is going away. And if mail is not picked up for a few days, someone should check with the elderly person to make sure they are okay.

Planning Early

It is beneficial for any person, no matter how young or old, to have an Emergency Plan of Action in place. It is essential that you have such a plan in place for your elderly parents, for a senior you care for, or an ill elderly person. The following is a list of things you should have in place in case of an emergency, but you should add to it to fit your specific situation. Look at it as a blue-print for your Emergency Plan.

EMERGENCY PLAN OF ACTION:

1. Durable Power of Attorney for health care and financial forms. Discuss the various options with your parent. This is to be done before a crisis occurs or signs of dementia present themselves.

2. Keep telephone numbers of your parent's physicians readily available.

3. Be sure to meet you parent's doctors and caregivers. If this is not possible in person, then speak to them by phone.

4. Make copies of your parents' Medicare card, Social Security card, all insurance cards, and insurance documents, and keep them with you.

5. Keep a current and accurate list of your parent's medications and instructions of use.

6. Establish which sibling is nearest to the parent and able to reach them first in a time of emergency. Make sure he or she has the above information.

7. Familiarize yourself with assisted living, residential care facilities, nursing homes, and home care agencies in your parent's neighborhood or your neighborhood. Consider where you parents can stay for a short time after a hospital stay so you are not caught off guard if the need occurs.

It would be wise to create a financial and legal plan early on, when your parent can be part of the planning. His or her wishes can be expressed then, making it easier on you knowing that you are fulfilling your parent's wishes. A plan that includes financial decisions should be in place.

The preplanning of financial provisions for the later years of one's life also minimizes the taxation on one's estate. Some of the taxes can be avoided by transfer of money to children years before long-term care is sought, and this way your parent may qualify for Medicaid, which will pay for long-term care in a nursing home or at the patient's house.

At the time that you are planning the future with your parent, you should check if there is long-term insurance in place. In the chapter on long-term insurance, you will find information on availability and cost of such insurance. The later in life you buy such insurance, the higher the cost.

As I said before, it is wise to plan ahead, before a crisis occurs, so that decisions are not forced upon us, and our options are not limited. The following are descriptions of the two main stages of crises we may encounter as our parents age:

Crisis I

The initial stages creep up almost unnoticed. Your parent starts slipping in behavioral and physical functions. It is a slow decline that can take months, even years, and is camouflaged in the beginning by the elderly. In general, the person seems to be doing okay. All too often, nobody pays attention to the fine signs when this is occurring.

Signs to look for:

a. Deterioration of personal hygiene

b. Unpaid bills, unopened mail

c. Carpets stained with food

d. Trouble remembering recent events

e. Changes in eating habits

f. Misplacing objects

g. Inability to remember if medication was taken or not

h. Unexplained bruises

i. Frequent calls to you or others

Crisis II

During this stage, signs of an escalation of symptoms are presented. It becomes clear not only to the professional caregivers, but also to family members that the level of care and involvement must be increased. This is a scary period, for us and for our loved ones, because it reminds us of our mortality. We also question our ability to rise to the task. But we will, if the need arises. And if our parents are able to perceive our love and sense our caring, it reassures them and provides them with a sense of security. Thus, it is very important that we show them care and love. At this stage, your parent is unable to deny or cope with the following:

a. Odors in the house

b. Urine stained carpet

c. Noticeable weight gain or loss

d. Skin tears or bruises

e. Repetitive phone calls at odd times

f. Inability to recall how the day was spent

g. Offensive mouth odor

h. Medication bottles either too full or too empty

i. Final notices on bills

j. Unexplained dents on the car.

This is the time that children cannot ignore the situation anymore and will have to step in. Early planning gives both you and your parents' control of the situation.

At this time you may consider moving the aging parent to live near you. This allows the parent to remain independent while you are near enough to help with their needs and with minimal disruption to your life. Not all parents will agree to this move. But if they do, you should consider the following:

a. Will their health insurance follow them with the move?

b. Is the move financially doable for them and for you?

c. Will the move afford them a social life, and religious contact, if they are used to those routines where they are currently living?

d. Is the climate suitable for them in the new place?

e. Will the new place afford them mobility? Are there stairs? Is there wheelchair access?

f. Will they feel safe?

Your parent should visit the potential residence before a decision is made and if possible should be included in the process of the decision-making.

Planning early for all eventualities allows you to evaluate each possibility for all the pluses and minuses they offer regarding your parent's specific needs. While researching the different options, it is best to take into account all components that may influence the decision of picking the right place to provide care for your parent.

One's religious needs, cultural needs, physical abilities, and language needs should be considered in any plan for long-term care. To find the most acceptable set up the parent should be part of the team that decides which solution is chosen. To make the parent part of the team, the process has to be initiated early, before signs of dementia are present.

That may not be so easy. If you approach your parents when they are in their sixties they may be taken aback, and, in all likelihood, they won't understand why you are thinking about such things so far in advance, when they are so active and independent.

It may be some time after you initially start the conversation before any inquiries or decisions are actually made. But it is smart to come back every so often to the topic, until your parents feel comfortable with the subject.

You must also consider that the fear is quite natural at this stage. Who wants to think about disabilities, physical and mental limitations, illnesses, partial or total dependency, and worst of all, mental inability to make any decisions pertaining to your life? Diplomacy is essential at this stage.

It may be much harder to start planning when the crisis is on hand, or your parent is unable to partake fully in the conversation. From my own experience dealing with my mother's issues, I realized that listening to our parents is a must for the outcome to be successful.

Case # 4

I first realized that it was time for me to step in after my father died and my mother suddenly was unable to make any kind of decision. She told my siblings and me, "You decide," and "I don't know what to do," regarding the simplest things, issues that just months ago she had dealt with on her own without anybody else's input.

She was resistant when we suggested that she sell her house. "Your father loved this house, it is my home," she countered. That the upkeep and the cost of running it would eat in to her savings made no difference to her. So we let her stay in her large house all by herself for the next 12 months. We let her write her own checks for utilities, and do her own banking. My mother had never done those things while my father was alive.

For the first few months she was proud of herself for running the house. But soon after she realized the extent of the expenses, and she began to see the rationale of selling her house.

Letting her come to that conclusion on her own, in her own time, was just right. This allowed her to feel that she was in control of her life, and that her children had not forced her to make those decisions.

This is true in many situations. When we were looking for an alternative living arrangement for my mother, she was part of the planning. Being that she was in her late seventies, fully alert, driving, and highly independent, she opted for an apartment, not far from my brother, where she still lives, though now with an aide 24/7.

You will find that when making such drastic decisions in the life of your parent or dear one, it makes a great difference if it is done with their participation and agreement. This makes it less dramatic for them and easier for you.

The Changing of Roles

At some point, as our parents age and become more and more dependent on us, our roles slowly reverse. We become the parents, and our parents become the children.

It is a process that varies from case to case. Some parents remain alert and active, into their late years. Others already become dependent on their children and relatives by their sixties. At times, this process takes longer, due to the fact that the children are reluctant to step in and take over the responsibility for directing care and making decisions.

The following points should be considered when your parent is aging and you are stepping in to help:

1. Write down all of your parents' financial assets, all of their insurance policies, real estate holdings, bank accounts, safe combinations. Familiarize yourself with the content of all documents. Make copies of all relevant documents, and place them in a different location, perhaps in your or your sibling's house, for safekeeping.

2. Make sure that all the original documents are kept in one place, and the place is known to you, or to someone else your parents trust.

3. Make sure that all documents that are time-sensitive are periodically updated. Make sure that a Living Will reflects your parents' wishes, and includes what should be done for them if they are unable to make decisions for themselves.

4. Encourage your parents to speak about, or to write down if it is easier, what their wishes are regarding the topic of funeral and burial. It may help to bring a third party into the equation: a friend, priest, rabbi,

a financial advisor, or other person. At times it is easier to express oneself to a stranger than to your child, regarding one's own death.

5. Make sure that you are aware of your parents' monthly expenses, and that they are paid on time. Elderly people commonly misplace bills, unopened bills or pay the same bill twice. As mentioned in the chapter on insurance, review the policies your parents have: life, health, car, or property insurance. Make sure that all policies are in effect, and that they cover whatever they are covering to the max. You may be surprised how many elderly people are paying for policies they no longer need.

In today's society, there are many families whose members live in different states, huge distances apart, and only some major calamity brings the children or relatives together to reluctantly step in and take control.

During the process of role reversal, the person assuming responsibility should consider the following:

1. Dealing with the new responsibility.

2. Incorporating that responsibility into your daily life.

3. Asking the parents' permission to be involved in their health issues.

4. Maintaining a dialogue with your parent regarding their living situation, and health and financial issues.

5. Trying to become a friend or a partner, but not a parent to your parents. They will cooperate with you to a greater degree if they do not perceive you treating them like children.

6. Being part of the solution, not the problem.

7. Involving other siblings or relatives in care-giving. Coordinating the sources of care so that there are no contradictions and the actual caregiver is not confused.

8. Never making unfair promises, such as "I will never put you in a nursing home," etc.

9. Evaluating options early.

To become the one responsible for your parent's or loved one's care is not an easy task. You, like all of us, have responsibilities of your own. You may have a family depending on you for care and support. You may still have young children. You may have an active career, which demands most of your waking hours. To direct your parent's daily life is not at all what you are looking for. But sometimes, this is what reality throws at us.

If it becomes necessary for you to take over the decision-making and to direct the care of your parent, it is important that you are emotionally accepting of this responsibility, instead of carrying resentment that will cause you to feel burdened and unhappy.

You should allow your loved one to do for him or herself as much as he or she can, for as long as she or he can. Be supportive of their efforts; do not criticize them for not doing things perfectly, or for making errors.

Reassure them that they can continue doing great on their own, with your help. You can review their bills, help them with writing checks, and check legal papers, such as lease renewals, insurance policies, etc. But it is important to maintain an atmosphere of being equals.

Think for a minute, if you were in need of help, and the person giving it to you were talking down to you, you would feel incompetent, helpless, maybe stupid for not being able to do the task on your own. This may be what your loved one feels. For the fear of negative feelings, many times our elders will not ask for help from their children and will continue to make mistakes, costly ones at times. They also do not want to be a burden, and do not want to lose control of their affairs. It is essential that you maintain a positive attitude toward your parent and encourage them to think positively.

When you reach the point that you need to take over the full care of your parent or dear one, you should do so with respect and appreciation of their situation. In most cases, the person you are stepping in to help is the one who gave you life, cared for you, and was there for you when you were sick, when you learned to ride a bike, or when you failed a test. Now it is your turn. So as inconvenient as it may be, you need to be there for them.

Even as the roles of parent and child reverse themselves in later years, we can carry out the task, while continuing to recognize the fact that they are our parents. We should not make them feel childish, that they are unable to care for themselves.

We should promote a sense of dignity and self-respect in our parents and help them to know that their life is of value even though they may need help from others to maintain their everyday routines.

Case # 5

My father was a teenager when World War II broke out in Eastern Europe. My mother was all of 14 years old, at the time. They met in a labor camp in the Ural Mountains. My father was caught by the Russian army while escaping the Germans in the Warsaw Ghetto, after his parents and younger siblings were shipped to a concentration camp where they were murdered.

My mother was separated from her mother, and wandered around the countryside unable to find her way home. She too was caught and sent to the same labor camp that my father was in.

Both worked in coal mines, pushing carts full of coal. One cart rolled backward, and hit my mother's back, causing her to suffer from damaged disks all her life. Her condition has deteriorated greatly over the years. My mother now has a morphine pump implanted inside her body to control her pain, allowing her to maintain some level of normalcy in her daily life.

My parents immigrated to the United States to improve and secure their lives and their children's lives. My whole family has loved living in this country and has taken pride in being American. My parents worked until their retirement, rather late in their lives. My siblings and I are working and paying into the system.

In his senior years, my father developed Parkinson's disease, which eventually killed him. He required expensive medication, costing hundreds of dollars per month, to deal with the debilitating symptoms and to reduce the demobilizing and demoralizing effects.

The cost of the treatments, medication, and home care completely wiped out all my parents' savings. My siblings and I helped as much as we could, but it is not easy to allocate part of your income to such expenses when you have your own family's needs to cover.

My father was lucky to have his children living fairly nearby and able to share the responsibilities of his care, both monetarily and physically. Although my father was a very proud man, we managed with much love and sensitivity to provide the care he needed, without making him feel needy. After his passing, we all realized that we were the lucky ones, for being there for my father when he needed us most.

Chapter 2 –
Government Health Related Programs
Know the Facts and Your Rights

Medicare:

In 1965, the government established the Health Insurance Program (Title XVII), which later became known as Medicare. Medicare is a federal program that is offered to every American over the age of 65. It is available to everyone, regardless of their financial status. But Medicare can be very confusing, for it offers a range of different plans. You qualify for Medicare regardless of whether you are already receiving Social Security, pensions of any kind, or disability. And you qualify for Medicare regardless of your assets. Medicare will also cover people under the age of 65 if they qualify, for example, because of disability.

On the official Medicare site, www.medicare.gov, you will find a great deal of information regarding the different programs and plans, and how you may qualify. The following summary may help you to evaluate the options.

When evaluating any of the Medicare plans, consider your personal situation and how Medicare will serve you. Here are some plans for your consideration:

Traditional Medicare:

This program is divided into two parts, Part A and Part B. Part A covers hospitalization and Part B covers medical payments, such as doctors. For Part B, you may pay through deductions from your Social Security monthly payment, or pay on your own, either directly or through health insurance that you carry. Both Part A and Part B pay partial payment on your cost for medical expenses and hospital costs.

Medicare covers about 80 percent of medical costs and hospital care. But it does not cover long-term care, such as a nursing home, or home care at the patient's home. It covers some rehabilitation, and short-term stays in long-term institutions. Many nursing homes are now developing subspecialties to increase income. So if a patient requires rehabilitation after hospitalization, and they qualify under Medicare, they can receive it in a long-term facility.

The following are some of the services covered under Medicare Part A:

- Laboratory work
- Home health services
- Hospice care
- Hospital stays
- Skilled nursing facility care

You should check the number of days covered for different services, and under what conditions the coverage is provided. For example, for hospice services, one needs to be terminally ill and expected to live no more then six months. The person can be recertified for an extension of another six months.

Medicare Part D:

The new Part D Medicare provides for a co-pay for your medication. There is a great deal of dissatisfaction with this program. First, it is fragmented; it is split between many HMO (Health Management Organization) insurance companies.

The medications they will cover differ from one HMO to another, which keeps the elderly and poor in a constant struggle to have prescriptions filled, which sometimes means changing insurance companies often.

The Part D program is a very complicated program that few of us understand. There are differences from one insurance company to the next, though each of them is under contract with Medicare to provide the medication to the Medicare member. Those insurance companies make the decision of whether and how much medication a patient will receive, even though their doctor already prescribed it. There are no statistics at this time as to the percentage of refusal to fill prescriptions for the elderly, but I am sure it is high.

There is a co-pay, which changes from one member of Medicare to another. My mother's plan has a co-pay of $1, $2, and $3. Yet every time she comes for her medication, the amount changes.

Some medications, such as some antibiotics, are refused on a regular basis, which requires the prescribing physician to call and make a special request, or in other words, justify the prescription. This is totally unacceptable. The doctor is forced to justify the need for the patient to receive a medication to some bureaucrat with no medical education, whose goal is to cut costs for the insurance company. Doctors are very unhappy to have to make those calls, for the simple reason that it takes hours to stay on the phone, with recorded messages and uncooperative telephone staff, trying to reach someone with authority who can get the right medication approved.

From my own experience, when my mother had a bout with pneumonia, the insurance company refused to fill her prescription for an antibiotic. When I spoke to them, they explained that they knew the drug to be ineffective- the person telling me this was not a doctor, not a nurse, but a secretary!

My mother has a thyroid condition. Her Medicare HMO refused her the medication Synthroid, which is the most widely used medication for her condition; the explanation was "the medication won't solve her problem; it will just improve her symptoms." Some of these insurance representatives have never dealt with medical issues, nor have they dealt with the elderly and sick. To them this is just a lucrative contract.

So, it is advisable to carefully compare the available insurance under the Part D Medicare program to make sure they cover yours, or your parent's medical needs, and that you will be able to receive the medication when you are in need of it.

Medicare provides you with coverage for medication, but it is not full coverage; you will still need additional insurance coverage, so as not to deplete your savings. Secondary insurance is available; the State Office of the Aged can be helpful in finding supplementary insurance in your state (see the information at the end of this book or on our website www.goldenyearsgolden.com).

Under Medicare Part D, people with limited income and resources may benefit from the help in paying for some health and prescription drug costs. Medicare also may qualify you for extra help, such as a low-income subsidy, to pay for your prescription drugs if your annual income (as of 2007) is below $15,315 if you are single, or $20,535 if you are married with a spouse and no other dependents. These amounts will change as of 2009.

If you qualify for extra help, you will receive help in paying your Medicare drug plan's monthly premium. Depending on your income and resources, you may have a reduced premium or no premium at all.

You may qualify for full Medicaid benefits, as well as receive Supplemental Security Income (SSI) benefits without Medicaid. SSI benefits are a monthly amount paid by Social Security to people with limited income and resources who are disabled, blind, or aged 65 and older. SSI benefits provide cash for basic needs, such as food, clothing, and shelter. SSI is separate from Social Security benefits.

To meet the conditions for receiving SSI benefits, you need to be a resident of the United States or the Northern Mariana Islands. You may not be absent for more than 30 days from the U.S., you must be either a U.S. citizen or in one of the categories of non-citizens. People who live in Puerto Rico, the Virgin Islands, Guam, or American Samoa may not get SSI. To find out if you or your parent qualifies for SSI, you may call 1-800-772-1213, or you can go to www.socialsecurity.gov.

Medigap

Medigap is an additional insurance option to cover the gaps between the Medicare insurance and the cost of medical care. There is a cost to such insurance, but in the long run it may protect your savings.

The "Doughnut Hole:"

The "doughnut hole," is the drug coverage gap between $2,250 and $5,100 in yearly out of pocket costs. Simply it means that your Medicare Part D will cover your prescription drugs up to $2,250. After that, you are responsible for the cost of the medication, until your expenses reach $5,100, at which time the insurance company steps in again to pay for your medication. This was created as a political compromise, but it affects millions of elderly; with the high cost of medication, they quickly fall into the gap, at times forced to choose between purchasing food and medication.

To eliminate the "doughnut hole" would cost our government a mere $5 billion, which would be just slightly over one percent of the total Medicare expenditure. This would not put a great burden on the government, and would be of untold benefit to the elderly, keeping them healthier, without the need to reduce or eliminate their medication because they cannot pay for it.

Investing in the improvement of Medicare Part D would be the proper and ethical thing for our society to do. This would help take care of the elderly, and at a cost that is a drop in the bucket, if you look at the general picture of government spending.

Qualified Medicare Beneficiaries (QMB)

This program is geared towards Specified Low-Income Medicare Beneficiaries (SLMB) to help with premiums, deductibles, and co-payments, for low-income people who are enrolled in the Medicare program.

Medicare covers some treatments, such as dialysis, which most of us don't realize. For someone who qualifies with low income assets, Medicaid will step in where Medicare will not cover the medical needs of that person.

To summarize, Medicare consists of two parts, Part A and Part B:

Part A covers most hospital bills, and some short-term nursing home stays, such as rehabilitation. Every person in America (American citizen or legal resident) is entitled to Medicare coverage; some may have slightly higher co-pays.

Part B provides Medicare participants with insurance for doctors' fees, but not for annual checkups. Some medical equipment, diagnostic tests, and outpatient care, as well as some mental care, are provided by Medicare. Short-term rehabilitative services are also covered. Most of the services mentioned here require a co-pay.

Most people pay approximately $90 as a monthly premium. The premium is deducted directly from their Social Security monthly payment. As of 2007, the monthly premium is linked to a person's income, i.e. the higher the income, the higher the premium.

People need a better understanding of the Medicare system. Seniors are being offered, by deceptive insurance agents, Medicare Advantage (MA) policies, which in most cases cover the same expenses that their old Medicare covered. Many of the elderly who sign up for these policies do not understand the Medicare Advantage plans, nor do they need them.

Thousands of seniors have fallen victim to illegal or unethical hard-sell tactics to sell them plans that often cover the same expenses they had through traditional Medicare; in the worst of scenarios, these plans may cost less, but not cover what the senior needs and have many more restrictions, especially on doctors and hospitals.

Some of these insurance agents have told seniors that the original Medicare has been closed, or is in the process of closing, so they should sign quickly or they will lose their coverage. One has to be very careful and suspicious of any insurance agent who is pushing and rushing you to sign on to their plan.

Out of the approximately 43 million people who are covered under Medicare, about 7 million have Medicare Advantage plans. For some it may be a good plan. But if one is coerced into signing up for a plan they don't actually need, it can be disastrous for their health and their financial situation.

Often seniors are not aware that they have switched an HMO until they need hospital services or a specialist. And when a senior tries to leave that HMO, it is very difficult and time-consuming.

There have been reports of people who tried to withdraw from such plans and were told that they could not. At the end of every year, between November 15 and December 31, you can choose to either withdraw, join another Medicare Advantage Plan, or remain enrolled in the one you are currently in. It is possible to change plans midyear if you have a reason to do so, but it is not easy.

If you are a senior citizen, you are in all likelihood bombarded with direct mail or phone calls encouraging you to join Advantage Medicare insurance programs.

It seems you cannot even watch television these days without a commercial promoting a Medicare program and making it hard to make an educated decision.

It is illegal for anyone to come to your home to sell you Medicare insurance if you did not invite them. If anyone comes and tells you that they are from Medicare, they are misrepresenting themselves. Tell them to leave immediately.

If you need to sort out which Medicare is appropriate for you and what each plan covers, go to www.medicare.gov or call 800-633-4227.

Do not be pushed into signing on to a plan immediately. Take a few days to think it over. If you have any questions, call and ask; if the insurance representative is unresponsive or seems to be unwilling to be clear and precise, the plan is not for you. Within the dates specified, you have the time to make your decision without being rushed.

I would suggest that you write out your specifics, such as the particular illness you have, and the medications you need. List the doctors that you use on a regular basis. Then check each program that you are considering. Are your doctors part of that network? Does the program provide your specific medication free of charge, at a minimal charge, or will you be required to pay higher fees for the medications you need?

You should also check if the particular insurance company that you are considering will limit the amount of the medication you need. Will you be required to constantly recertify the medication prescribed by your doctor?

Once you find the Medicare program that is best suited for you, call your primary doctor and ask him or her if that particular program is one that they accept and recommend. The doctors are the ones who have a great deal of experience dealing with the insurance companies and are very knowledgeable as to which are easiest to deal with.

Pointers:

Medicare Part A: Covers Hospital Insurance
Medicare Part B: Covers Medical Insurance

* Medicare provides the above coverage.

* You have your choice of doctors.

* Generally, Medicare Part B pays 80% of covered costs and you pay 20%, after you meet your deductible.

Medicare Part C: Includes both part A and B

* Private insurance companies are approved to provide this coverage.
* In most plans you will have to see the plan's doctors.
* You will have to pay co-payments in most cases for covered services.
* Costs, extra benefits, and rules may vary from plan to plan.

Proscription Drug Coverage Part D

* To be eligible for this program you need to be a subscriber of Medicare.
* You must join a Medicare Prescription Plan.
* Plans are run by private insurance companies that are approved by Medicare.
* Most Medicare Advantage Plans usually include prescription drug coverage for an extra cost.

Supplemental Coverage:

* You can choose to purchase private supplemental coverage.
* Costs may vary from one company to another, as well as one policy to another.
* Employers, as well as unions, may offer similar coverage.
* You may want to supplement your coverage with private coverage.

It is wise to check with your local Medicare office whether you need supplemental insurance and if you can keep it under your Medicare plan.

Special Needs Plan (SNP):

The Special Needs Plan serves people who live in an institution, such as a nursing home, or any other long-term facility, or are eligible for both Medicare and Medicaid. People who qualify for the SNP may have one or more specific chronic or disabling conditions, such as diabetes, congestive heart failure, mental illness, HIV, or AIDS.

This program provides Medicare prescription drug coverage. In some cases a care coordinator will be required to help you develop a personal care plan.

SNP manages the services provided to you to keep you healthy and help you follow your doctor's instructions. You need to check if your doctor accepts Medicare and Medicaid for the services he or she provides.

To clarify what you are eligible to receive from your Medicare coverage, call the Medicare office for their MEDICARE & YOU BOOKLET; it will guide you in making the right decision. For more information go to www.medicare.org.

Make sure that you review the cost, coverage, and convenience of your current plan, compare it with other plans in your area, and check if you may be better off with a different plan. If you are happy and satisfied with the plan you are in, you need not do anything; your coverage will continue through the next year.

Between November 15 and December 31 you can change your Medicare health or prescription coverage for the coming year. If you made a change, your new coverage will begin on January 1.

Medicare offers a great deal of literature that covers all possibilities, and they offer phone support to help you navigate through their system and make the right decisions. For contact information go to www. medicare.org.

Medicaid

Medicaid is a federal program that provides assistance with medical expenses to low-income people regardless of age. If you or your parent qualifies for Medicaid, you will be satisfied that between Medicare and Medicaid and you do not need additional coverage.

Basically, Medicaid is a public welfare program. The program covers what Medicare does not. Medicaid will cover custodial care in the patient's home or in a nursing home, for people who can't afford it and whose doctor recommends such assistance.

Most of us assume that this program is not for us, but with the current regulations, you would be surprised who qualifies.

Not only do some middle-class people qualify for the program, but some fairly wealthy people have even squeezed into it as well, thanks to legal loopholes, by virtue of establishing trusts, gifts, annuities, and other ways to transfer wealth to kids and family members. All you need is a shrewd and well-informed lawyer.

As of last year, the system has become more challenging to navigate, and some of the loopholes have been eliminated. As with any governmental program, you need to check the rules and regulations annually, for they do change. Qualifying numbers go up and down, and although your parent may qualify this year, they may not qualify next year.

It is important to be familiar with the spending policies of Medicaid, to protect whatever assets you can. It is a good idea to consult an attorney specializing in this field, such as an elder law attorney.

If you are single and entering a nursing home, you will, in all probability, have to sell your home and devote all of your assets to covering the cost of the nursing home care. Once the money is gone, the nursing home will qualify you for Medicaid. After that, Medicaid will pay for your care for the rest of your life. If you gave your money away to your heirs in the few years before qualifying for the care, Medicaid may penalize you and not cover you for a period of time. However this decision can be appealed.

If you are married, and only one of the spouses is entering a nursing home, the rules of the assets may change. First, the spouse staying at home will not be forced to sell the house. According to a recent *Newsweek article by* Jane Bryant Quinn, such items as furniture, auto, and life insurance, some savings, in the range of $20,328 to $101,640 (depending on the state in which you live), can remain in the possession of the spouse remaining at home.

In many cases, spouses split finances, so as not to jeopardize all their possessions when one of them has to be moved to a nursing home. If one pays initially from his or her savings for nursing home care, it may allow him or her to choose a better nursing home. Once the assets in his or her name are depleted, Medicaid steps in to pick up the bill until the end of the patient's life.

So it is advisable for couples to plan ahead.

If you seek Medicaid coverage for care and services, you will have to submit proof of your resources.

Upon applying for Medicaid, you will be asked to choose one of the following:

1. Community coverage **without long-term care,**
2. Community coverage **with** community based long-term care
3. Medicaid coverage for **all options**

To receive Medicare and Medicaid information, visit or call your local Social Security office. Information can be mailed to you, or if you are disabled, you can request that an information agent visit you at home.

The following is general information on what services are covered and what the requirements to qualify for Medicaid are.

Community Coverage Without Long-Term Care

This coverage, if one qualifies, will be suitable for a person who does not need nursing facility services or community based long-term care. In other words, if you qualify, you will receive Medicaid coverage for all services except nursing home care. You need to present all required financial documentation to prove your need.

Those who document their financial resources, including income and savings, according to the regulations in their state, may be eligible for short-term rehabilitation services. Short-term rehabilitation provides only one admission in a period of 12 months. The rehabilitation will be provided for a maximum of 29 consecutive days. This service is provided in certified institutions.

Community Coverage With Community Based Long-Term Care

This includes the following services:

a. Adult day health care
b. Limited licensed home care
c. Certified home health agency services

    d.   Hospice in the community

    e.   Hospice residence program

    f.   Personal care services

    g.   Personal emergency response services

    h.   Private duty nursing

    i.   Residential treatment facility

    j.   Consumer directed personal assistance program

    k.   Assisted living program

    l.   Managed long term care in the community

    m. Home and community-based services waiver program

To qualify for the above services through Medicaid, you will need to fill out their application, which asks about all of your financial resources. If you should later require nursing home services, Medicaid will examine your financial resources for up to 36 months in the past.

Medicaid Coverage for All Covered Care and Services

This includes the following:

    a.   Nursing home care

    b.   Nursing home care provided in hospital

    c.   Home and community-based waiver services

    d.   Hospice in a nursing home

    e.   Managed long-term care in a nursing home

    f.   Intermediate care facility

For one to be eligible for the services above the financial resources will be checked for up to 36 months back; trust accounts, up to 60 months back. This is to be done before the application is filed. If you are found to be eligible, you will be covered for all Medicaid services.

The local Department of Aging assists the elderly with Medicaid forms and billing problems, and will be able to provide you with lists of participating health care providers. For contact information of the

Department of Aging in your state, check the back of this book or visit our website www.goldenyearsgolden.com .

Other Benefits:

Supplemental Security Income (SSI)

Among other benefits available to a person in need is Supplemental Security Income (SSI). If you are certified blind or disabled, age 65 or older, and your income and resources are below certain limits, you may be eligible for SSI. You can apply for SSI at your local Social Security office. Most people who receive SSI also receive medical assistance.

Interim Assistance

You may be eligible for Interim Assistance financial aid through the Family Assistance/Safety Net Assistance Program, if you:

1. Applied for SSI but your application has not been approved or denied.
2. You are appealing a suspension of your SSI.
3. Your SSI has been stopped.

Home Energy Assistance Program (HEAP)

This program can help you with heating and utility costs and certain essential heating equipment repairs. You may be able to receive Home Energy Assistance if:

1. You already receive temporary assistance.
2. You already receive the Food Stamps benefit.
3. You already receive SSI.
4. Your income is at or below current guidelines.
5. You live in subsidized housing and pay directly for heating costs.

As with all federal and state programs, nothing is written in stone, and rules and regulations may change yearly, or with changes of administrations. So make sure that you keep up to date on information.

To find out if you qualify for assistance, check with the appropriate offices, or with the Office of the Aging in your state, for which contact information can be found at the end of this book.

Social Security-
How secure are we that it will be there for us.

Social Security came into existence in 1935, signed into being by President Roosevelt. At the time of its creation, there were no facilities, no staff and no budget. The initial personnel were loaned to the Social Security Administration, originally called the Social Security Board, from other federal agencies. In the first ten years the program went through several name changes and reorganizations.

Originally, President Roosevelt commissioned a group to develop a comprehensive program for social insurance that would cover all major personal economic hazards, with emphasis on unemployment and old age insurance. From that plan the Bureau of Federal Old-Age Insurance was developed, eventually becoming the Social Security program we know today.

In July of 1946 the agency was formally named Social Security Administration, with Arthur Altmeyer as its first Commissioner. The vastness of the Title II Program (Old Age Benefits) had required considerable decentralization. At the initial stage there were 12 regional offices, with new regional offices constantly opening over time. In 1973, the Bureau of Supplemental Security Income (SSI) was established.

According to the 2007 Trustees Report, 49 million people were receiving benefits from the program by the end of 2006. Among the recipients were 34 million retired workers and their dependents, and seven million disabled workers and their dependents. During the same year, 162 million people paid payroll taxes into Social Security. In 2006, $546 billion were paid in benefits, and $745 billion were collected. Currently Social Security has assets of about $2 trillion that are held in special issued U.S. Treasury securities.

Some sources state that with the senior population growing, the birth rate decreasing, people living longer, and benefits being paid out for more years than ever before, the payout of benefits will be greater than the amount of dollars coming in. Economists predict that the difficulties in funding the payout benefits will manifest themselves in 10 to 20 years.

The Social Security program will touch virtually every American in the future, assuming that it survives. Every few years we are reminded that the program will go under in 15, or 20, or 40 years; whatever the prediction, it is clear that the program is in trouble. Meanwhile, it continues to make the lives of many of our seniors easier.

Now, with the influx of millions of baby boomers, the system will become even more stressed, not only due to possible fiscal issues, but also due to inherent problems in the administration of the program. The physical acceptance of new cases will become more difficult due to the shortage of personnel. With all the cuts and down-sizing of staff, people applying for Social Security benefits have a longer wait ahead of them.

Especially worrisome is the fact that new applications for disability cases are delayed in processing or in the setting up of hearing dates, all due to shortage of staff. Although the Social Security Administration has about 1500 offices throughout the country that provide services to Americans reaching the qualifying age, or applying for disability, that number is not high enough to accommodate all the requests with which they are inundated.

In small towns the wait to be seen by a Social Security administrator may be hours, or in some cases days or weeks. And the wait is much longer to see a judge in a disability case. Since the 1970s the workforce in the offices of Social Security has been shrinking.

With stricter security laws, all employers will be required, under the penalty of law, to check Social Security cards and verify their authenticity. This will require increased hours for Social Security administration personnel.

As stated before, the demands on the Social Security administration increase, and their labor force decreases, we can expect to see even longer lines in their offices, and much longer waiting periods for issues that we have to be resolved. There are complaints not only from people in need of Social Security services, but also from the Social Security employees who are overwhelmed by the increased workload.

The Social Security administration's budget has been cut by the Bush administration (2000 and 2008) as well as by Congress. Senator

Kent Conrad, chairman of the Senate Budget Committee, has said that his committee recommended that Social Security be appropriated $430 million above the president's request for the agency for the year 2008.

As of September 2007, the first baby boomer began applying for Social Security benefits. If many of the new retirees apply using the Internet, the process will be easier and faster. However, considering the aging computerized systems currently used by the Social Security administration, it will still take longer than if the equipment were more up-to-date. For the seniors, and those who are about to become seniors, this may be the most important governmental agency that they deal with, or will deal with in the future. Let's hope that the agency is ready for them.

To reach the social security offices, call toll-free: 1-800-772-1213 or visit www.ssa.gov.

Chapter 3 –
The Different Residential Options & Cost

Considering the Different Residential Options:
Take a deep breath...

There comes a time when a decision needs to be made regarding setting up a residential situation for your loved one or yourself, if staying on your own is no longer an option.

You should review all the options presented in this chapter. Visit as many different residential situations as you can before you make your decision.

Making the Right Decision

Here are some of the choices:

YOUR HOME

Most people will agree that the best of all choices is to live for as long as possible in one's own home. There should be, of course, proper conditions for safety. If your parent's or loved one's health status allows, I fully recommend that he or she continue to live at home.

Polls show that 89 percent of people older than 50 would like to stay in their home and maintain their independence for as long as they possibly can. With the many technical aides that exist today, and new devices that are being developed at a very fast pace, staying at home has become easier.

The most popular devices that people currently have in their homes are blood pressure and sugar level monitoring units. If the reading is abnormal, they can immediately seek medical advice. Additionally, an emergency button, connected to a central office, will alert the center for immediate help when the button is pressed.

As the ability of the elderly to care for him or herself diminishes, and their safety is jeopardized, home care can be introduced, thus allowing the senior to continue to stay in his or her home for much longer.

There are agencies that will step in on an as-needed basis to provide care of the home, cleaning, laundry, and shopping, which can be provided as little as a few hours a week. Agencies that provide these services tend to be slightly less expensive than licensed and certified home-care services.

There are currently more then 8,000 home-care agencies that are certified for provision of services for Medicare and Medicaid, quite a few thousand of which that are licensed throughout the United States. Licensed agencies can contract with certified agencies and provide home care for patients on Medicare and Medicaid.

The next step is when the person requires a higher level of care. If their mobility is affected, if they are unable to go to their doctor on their own, if they are unable to dress themselves, bathe on their own, or cook for themselves, they will require home care. But even then, home care can be provided for them in 4- or 8-hour increments, a few days a week, and additional hours can be added as needed, eventually becoming day and night care.

When looking for an agency that provides home care, you need to check that the agency is licensed by the state it is in, and that it is in good standing. The state office of home care will be able to give you this information. Ask for client recommendations; no agency will refer you to a client that is unhappy with their services, but you still can get a great deal of information from them. The length of time the client has been using the agency can be a key. No one who is unhappy with the service will use the agency for an extended time.

If it is a licensed agency, and you should only use a state-licensed or certified agency, it should comply with all rules, laws, and regulations required by state and federal agencies.

A licensed agency has met all requirements of the state department of health, hires only legal residents of this country who are trained and qualified as Home Health Aides (HHA) or Personal Care Aides (PCA), and are overseen by a Registered Nurse (RN).

Most licensed agencies will also provide a wide range of services, such as physical therapy, occupational therapy, social services, etc. Such agencies must, by law, carry all relevant insurance coverage, such as liability, workmen's compensation, and disability, and they are bonded.

A certified agency is a licensed agency that becomes certified for the purpose of contracting for services paid for by the government. So to be able to bill Medicaid and Medicare for services, an agency has to be certified. When I had my agency, there was a moratorium in place in my state; thus our agency was unable to be certified by the state and bill the government directly. This precluded us from taking any patients who had Medicaid and/or Medicare coverage.

There is, however, a way to bypass the moratorium by contracting with a certified agency, and in fact becoming a vendor for them. So the patient in need of home care is actually serviced by a licensed agency that bills the certified agency, which in turn bills Medicaid for the services.

The certified agency takes a small cut per hourly fee, and passes on the contracted hourly fee to the licensed agency. Most of the time the nursing services, such as weekly visits, etc., are also provided by the certified agency.

This should not make a difference to the patient, except when there are problems with workers or coverage, on holidays and weekends, or when agencies are usually closed. In times like this, you may be forced to deal with two agencies, with one agency sometimes transferring the responsibility to the other.

Both agencies use HHAs, but only licensed agencies will use PCAs.

HHAs have more extensive training, thus Medicaid only approves HHAs for their patients. Both HHAs and PCAs will assist or provide all levels of care, in activities of daily living (ADLs).

Home care services agencies are currently among the fastest growing businesses in the country. As more and more dollars are funneled into them from the government and insurance companies, there is a noticeable need to establish greater control and regulation for home care services, to protect patients.

The most noticeable item that is still missing is a registry of all home care aides that are licensed and registered with the given state. This is essential to protect the patient from fraudulent certification or license holders and people untrained in the field. Schools that provide training for HHAs should be better controlled and held responsible for their program and their standards for students' performances. The government needs to make sure that the patient that is in his or her home is protected and cared for by well-qualified aides.

A centralized registry with well kept accountability will be useful to weed out the unqualified aides, as well as keep track of aides who have been found negligent in their duties or of harming patients. This way if they are fired from one agency for wrongdoing, they will not be able to apply to a different agency that might be unaware of their history.

In New York State there are about 140 agencies that provide home care services. Some of them are quite large, providing services for more than 500 patients. Some are small, and serve 30 to 40 patients. All depend on the HHA to do their job well and provide the best services to the patient at home. But the supervision that these agencies provide differs from one to the other. One may think that the larger agencies provide better care for the elderly, but that may not necessarily be so. Some smaller agencies may provide more personable care and be more available to patients.

Some of the agencies are reachable 24 hours a day, 365 days a year. When you call on holidays or on a weekend, some agencies will have a recording asking you to leave a message describing your problem, and then someone will get back to you on the next business day.

When choosing an in-home service through a home care agency, call on weekends, nights, and holidays to see if there is a reliable support system. If you reach a recorded message, leave a message and ask to be called back, and see how long it takes. If you are not called back in 15 minutes, you should look for another agency. If you or your loved one has an emergency, you want to reach someone who is able to assist you or respond to you immediately.

Although there are many agencies that do not provide optimal services, most provide wonderful services and fill the gap that at one time was filled by family members, providing the care that allows many elderly and disabled people to remain in their own home. All you have to do is make sure that the agency you chose is one that provides this kind of care.

The best choice ensures that a disabled, ill, or elderly person is cared for by an aide and made to feel comfortable and safe in their own home. One stays in his or her home, among his or her belongings, in an environment they love and that carries with it memories and familiarity. What could be better?

A good agency will be tuned in to the personality needs of the client, such as language, culture, and religious preferences and practices. If the client is Jewish and keeps a kosher kitchen, the aide should be in-serviced on the topic, and be able to accommodate this practice in the client's kitchen.

An aide is not only there to assist the client with his ADLs, the aide is also a companion, who will stimulate social interaction and seek out social activities in the neighborhood which the client may enjoy. The aide will take the client to his or her appointments and do their shopping.

As the client ages, when mental as well as health status changes, it may become difficult for the elderly person to handle his or her finances and oversee daily spending. That's the time when a relative or a friend should step in and help.

It is very important that the agency and the aides are kept accountable for all that goes on in the client's home. Even if the agency does not practice it, you should demand that the aide keep a log where vital signs are recorded, as well as any changes in health. So if the client has not eaten well or slept well, the next aide will know about these changes. Also the nurse visiting the client will know how the week proceeded for the client.

Another log should be kept by the aide regarding financial issues. I always encouraged the family, friend, or guardian to give weekly expense money to the aide; the amount should be written into the log, and all expenses recorded and receipts kept, so all can be checked for accuracy, and the balance reflect the money left.

During my work in home care, I found that some relatives did not want to bother with the bookkeeping. But this is very important as it will keep the aide accountable and she or he will know that someone is "watching."

When the routines are established, home care flows easily. Everyone knows his role in the running of the household and the care of the client.

If you or your parents are determined to remain at home in later years, you may have to make some modifications to make the home safe. Many accidents can be avoided if the home accommodates the changes that are likely to occur with the aging process. Those changes may be physical, mental, or both. See the Chapter on Safety for the Elderly.

The cost for care given in the client's home can vary greatly from state to state, and even within the state from city to city. The cost per hour can be as low as $9 and as high as $25. If you need 24-hour coverage, the cost can range from $100 to $250. This is still cheaper than if the care were paid per hour for 24 hours. You will have to do good research and a comparison study to find the best agency with the best price.

If you decide to stay in your home, and if you have limited finances that won't last for a very long time, you may consider the reversed mortgage option. There are companies, and you may have seen their advertisements on television, that will qualify you, if you are 62 years or older. They will pay you monthly payments for as long as you live, even if the equity in your house is used up. After your passing, your house ownership is transferred to the mortgage company. Be aware that there are up-front fees, and it may vary from company to company.

Another option, though not often used, is to sell your home to someone, usually a family member, and rent it from them, thus providing you with the money that you need to live on and allowing you to remain in your own home. This type of arrangement can also be made with some charitable organizations. There may even be a tax benefit in it for your estate.

To reduce the cost of staying in your own home, you can also take in a boarder, someone who will pay you rent to live in your house. The upside is that the renter will be there for you in a time of emergency; the downside is that you lose some of your privacy, and you need to be considerate of someone else's needs. See the Shared Housing option later in this chapter.

Staying in your own home during your elder years has many benefits, as explained in this chapter, but you need to weigh the pros and cons for your specific situation.

ADULT DAY CARE

Adult Day Care is a center that provides activities during the day for the elderly. The arrangement provides a social environment, promoting interaction with others and thus avoiding isolation. Most centers are open five days per week. They provide social activities, and meals that are free or at a token fee. Some take trips and bring in lecturers on various topics that appeal to the elderly.

Some programs provide transportation to the centers and back home, making it easy for a person to attend. Some also provide health screenings, such as taking blood pressure, providing flu vaccinations, or checking blood sugar.

The centers are also good channels for identifying people who are falling by the wayside. Some of the centers have social workers visiting regularly and can be of help with getting Medicare and Medicaid, etc., for the client. If there is significant deterioration in the health or mental status of the elder, it is usually easily picked up by the staff of the center. The staff then notifies the family or the participant's doctor.

Most of these centers are funded by different government programs, or religious or philanthropic organizations. This allows most centers to be open to all elderly. It is likely that more and more such centers will be established.

If you have such a center in your neighborhood or the center you are interested in has transportation available for people who live a distance away, and you do not qualify for free services, you will find that private cost is fairly reasonable. Some of the centers we called cost no more than $50 per day, and provide services and care from 7:45 am until 4:30 pm. They also provide breakfast, hot lunch, and a snack.

In large cities, the cost for care in an adult day care center tends to be higher than in a smaller town. We found prices ranging from $50 per day, up to $185. Most include one or two meals; some have special programs for Alzheimer's clients, or memory-stimulating programs.

We also found that religious institutions, such as churches or synagogues that run adult day care programs tend to be less costly to the private payer. Those centers also provide a wider range of activities for their clients, and the staff is usually better trained than in the very small private centers. So you need to scrutinize the program before you make your choice, making sure that the adult day care center is licensed and the staff is trained in the care of the elderly and disabled.

Most long-term insurance will not cover adult day care, but as the senior population is growing, and as the baby boomers enter that stage, the demand for such coverage will grow. Fairly healthy adults may benefit from such an arrangement, and it will cost the insurance company much less than a stay at a nursing home or assisted-living facility.

If your parent lives with you, and you are fully employed and gone from the house most of the day, it may well be the best arrangement for your parent. He or she will be in a safe environment, provided one or two meals, remain socially engaged, and be stimulated mentally. This will unquestionably give you peace of mind during the day, not having to worry about them. Then when you pick up your parent, or he or she is brought home, you may spend quality time together. This kind of arrangement allows you to keep a normal routine in your personal life.

For information on how to locate adult day care centers, contact your state's Office of the Aged.

GOVERNMENT SUBSIDIZED SENIOR HOUSING
SECTION 202 HOUSING

Section 202 housing is administered by the Department of Housing and Urban Development (HUD). Most units in this type of housing are small, i.e. studios or one bedroom apartments. All units are designed for seniors and have built-in safety features, including no-skid floors, grab bars in the bathrooms, wide hallways, safety railings, elevators, and ramps.

The apartments are outfitted with emergency buttons, for personal safety; the communal spaces, such as laundry rooms, are geared towards people who are older. The spaces are well-lit, the washing machines and dryers are simple to operate. Transportation and shopping are also available for the seniors. In some buildings there are also provisions for meals.

To qualify for Section 202 housing, the candidate has to be at least 62 years old and with low income. The level of income changes slightly yearly, so you have to check with HUD for current numbers. One needs to be self-sufficient and able to live independently to qualify.

Statistics show that the majority of residents in this type of housing are women, over 70 years old, and with an income less than $10,000. The advantage of this option is that it is very affordable since the rent is very low, between $190 and $300 per month, which includes utilities, such as electricity and gas. The resident maintains his or her privacy and independence, while living in a safe environment.

The disadvantages are that the waiting lists for these apartments are long. It varies from state to state, and in some places, like New York, the wait is years. Many times while on the waiting list, the applicant's health status may change, making the apartment unsuitable for him or her.

This residential setting does not accommodate the frail and the elderly who are unable to care for themselves and their daily needs. So if you or your parent move into Section 202 housing, you need to understand that if health status changes and a higher level of care is required, you will have to move to an appropriate facility that provides that necessary care.

Overall residents are very content with this option. There is a built-in social environment by the sheer fact that all the residents are in the same age group. They all deal with the same issues, such as health, daily activities, limitations due to age, etc. The best part is the low cost of living in such a building.

This option should be made more available in the future. With the increase in the aging American population the demand for affordable housing will increase. With planning we can add services such as meals to all buildings, and make home care aides more available. This will eliminate the need to move the resident, unless he or she is very ill and requires more specialized care.

Such housing projects should be built into neighborhoods that offer shopping, parks, and health clinics to meet the needs of the elderly.

For more information regarding Section 202 housing contact your state's Office of the Aged.

ADULT FOSTER CARE

This type of care is provided in residential homes, and generally includes room and board, as well as assistance in daily activities, such as bathing, grooming, etc.

Residents of adult foster care are independent, but 24-hour private care is available, paid directly by the resident. If needed, the care giver can reside on the premises.

Adult foster care is an option for an individual who is fairly independent and can control and direct his or her needs. It is less costly than assisted living or retirement communities, and the services provided are very basic.

Adult foster care also varies in its range of services, and the number of residents it accommodates. In general these homes are not large, and accommodate as little as six or eight residents and up to twenty. Food is usually provided and served in a dining room, which promotes social interaction.

Laundry and cleaning services are available to its residents; room cleaning is also provided. Residents are free to come and go as they wish. The residents are responsible for their needs, other than room and board which they pay directly to the adult foster care. If a resident needs assistance in traveling to doctors' appointments or a beauty parlor appointment, the arrangement can be made through the caretaker in the adult foster care.

This arrangement is very much like living independently, but with the added security that someone will be there in a time of need. And it does make it easier not to have to worry about basic chores of everyday needs. This option is suitable for people who want easier routines and some social interaction, while not being in an overregulated environment.

To find more information on adult foster care, contact your state's Office of the Aged.

CONTINUING CARE

Continuing care retirement communities are being developed all over the country. In many cases, they incorporate independent living, assisted living, as well as nursing homes, all on the same site. This allows a resident to move from one type to another, as health, and physical status changes.

One thing that we should keep in mind while considering this option: the high price tag that is attached. As this "all-in-one" option takes hold, and becomes more popular, the financing of this possibility is becoming more and more creative, though it remains a high-ticket choice.

The entry fee can be $260,000, which is nonrefundable, or it can be as high as $350,000, part of which will be refundable if the person leaves the community or dies, in which case a portion of the down payment will be refunded to their heirs. Aside from the hefty entrance fee, there is a monthly maintenance fee of approximately $4,000.

Traditionally, the monthly fee remains the same, even if the level of care changes. But you should be careful and ensure this in writing. The rapid changes in the field of health care bring constant changes in cost, so be very careful when signing on the dotted line.

In the last few years, about 20 to 30 new communities have been built annually, and there are hundreds of creative plans for financing continuing care. Some of those communities charge higher prices upfront, and the monthly fee is lower. Others do the opposite.

Some of the continuing care centers will include in their maintenance fee only the cost for the basics, such as grounds, residential structure, communal areas, and recreational areas. All personal care, as well as health care, is provided based on individual need, and paid for directly by the recipient of the service.

This arrangement eliminates the cost of long-term insurance, since the continuing care facility includes higher levels of care. Higher maintenance fees paid now may cost more, but will save money in the future if nursing care is required.

The initial fee is essentially how much the unit that you are going to live in will cost you. In all likelihood it is priced higher than a comparable unit on the free market, but it costs more because services are also included.

Residents of such communities like the fact that they are homeowners. The switch from independent living is less traumatic when entering a continuing care community. It is not an institutionalized setting; it is a neighborhood.

Most of the continuing care communities provide a full range of services, such as laundry, food deliveries, dining services on the premises, all at the level of independent living. Residents can cook in their private kitchen, or eat meals in the communal dining room with other residents.

When researching the more than 900 continuing care communities, you can log on to www.ccrdata.org, which will direct you to the nearest community and list the services it provides as well as the costs.

There are a number of reasons to choose continuing care. You live at the independent level for as long as possible, and in time, if you need assistance with daily activities, you just move to the assisted living facility. And if you eventually need a higher level of care, you can move to the nursing home. All of these levels of residence are based in the same community. This allows for a smooth and easy transition.

This arrangement eliminates a common dilemma that people encounter: What will happen if I am unable to remain independent at home, or what if I cannot remain in assisted living because I need much more personal care? It is basically a place in which one can stay for life, enjoying all levels of living, and not worrying about the next level of need.

Sometimes long-term care insurance can be applied, even if it is partial payment. When purchasing a long-term insurance policy, check the coverage to see if it will apply for personal care in a continuing care situation.

For more information on Continuing Care Communities in your state, contact the Continuing Care Associations and Office of the Aging.

ASSISTED LIVING

As we age, illnesses, falls, and other circumstances may make it impossible for us to stay in our own homes. But for some of us remaining independent is very important. When that moment in life comes when we need to make a choice, due to the need for a greater support system, help with daily activities, or because of issues of safety, one of the options is an assisted living facility. The growing number of elderly Americans has contributed to the establishment of a range of residential options which cater to the elderly.

More than one million Americans are currently living in assisted living environments. Assisted living facilities are designed for people who are no longer able to live on their own, but want to maintain their independence for as long as they can.

It is important to research what services you or your parent need, and then make sure that the particular facility you are interested in can provide those services. For help in finding such facilities in your state check our website www.goldenyearsgolden.com .

Assisted living facilities are set up for higher functioning individuals. Most residents in assisted living facilities are people who are ambulatory and can partake in social and recreational activities, such as sports, games, parties, exercises, and educational sessions, etc. The population in such a facility is generally healthy, and when the residents' health deteriorates, they are encouraged to find other residential arrangements. Most of these facilities are not fully safety proofed.

In the last few years, some of the assisted living facilities have been built as part of a long term care complex, which includes a higher care facility; therefore when a resident of the assisted living requires greater care because of health problems, he or she can be transferred to a nursing home or related facility. But that kind of higher level of care is only available in some assisted living facilities.

Assisted living facilities mostly do not provide medical care (nursing homes do), but they do provide assistance with daily living activities, such as bathing, dressing and feeding. Those services can be provided and charged for on a daily, weekly, or monthly basis. This range of services can be provided for years, if no skilled medical and nursing care is needed.

Assisted living facility residents often have their own apartments or units. Meals are generally provided in common dining rooms, and support staff offer assistance with health care needs of daily living.

The following services are generally provided in most assisted living facilities:

* Help with eating, bathing, dressing and toileting (activities of daily living).
* Reminders to take medication.
* Monitoring and managing health care.
* Help with housekeeping and laundry.
* Range of recreational activities.

* Transportation to doctor's offices and shopping, etc.
* Security, in unit or apartments, personal safety, and general safety in the   facility and around it.

The typical resident of an assisted living facility is a 75-year old woman. This is due to the fact that women, in general, live longer than men. Many married couples also choose to live in assisted living facilities, and many units are set up to accommodate couples.

Assisted living facilities are for the most part high-end facilities. The common areas, such as dining rooms, recreational clubs, outdoor areas, hallways, entryways and lobbies, are usually quite elegant.   However, residents' rooms are at times quite a step down from what a visitor sees.

In some assisted living facilities residents are not required to take all their meals in common dining room. In some facilities residents will have a small kitchenette, where they can prepare their own meals. But it is encouraged that some meals be eaten in the dining room to reduce potential isolation.

If at all possible, bring your parent to visit such a facility, and speak to residents randomly, not just the ones that the facility provides. Wander around the facility; looking into residents' rooms without a representative of the facility, and visit floors that are not normally shown on tours for potential residents.

A social person who adapts quickly to new social situations tends to interact with others easily, and was previously very active and independent will adapt well to such a place. If your parent is withdrawn and shy, he will be lonely and isolated in such a facility. The staff tends to let residents set their own pace of participation in social activities, and if a resident chooses to sit in his or her room most of the hours of the day, no one will come to encourage them to join activities. For the most part, residents are left on their own.

If your parent likes to take walks, check if the facility's grounds can accommodate continuation of this healthy habit. If your parent liked to swim, make sure there is a swimming pool. It is important that he or she live the quality of life they had before becoming residents in an assisted living facility. If your parent has lived all of his or her life in an urban setting, it will be difficult to move to a suburban setting. But there are assisted living facilities in both urban and suburban areas.

Some of the facilities provide a range of services, such as help with bathing, and an aide if sudden illness occurs. But these services are not included in the monthly cost. Arrangements are made individually, and paid by the resident directly. At times such services are provided by an outside vendor, arranged outside the bureaucracy of the facility, and without the facility having any responsibility as to the quality of services provided by the agency.

Most such assisted living facilities are geared to single occupancy, but double rooms are available too. Double rooms can produce another set of problems. Personality match is essential for maintaining a peaceful and friendly everyday life, much as in a college dorm.

Each state has different regulations and licensing requirements, which you should check in to, to ensure that the facility is complying with all the state health department requirements and has the required license. You can also check with the health department and the State Office of the Aged for the safety record of the specific facility.

If the facility has no safety features in the residents' rooms, such as safety bars in the bathroom, easy-to-open locks on doors, good lighting in the room, bathrooms, and hallways, as well as a stall shower to make it easy to step in and out of a shower, you can negotiate for those needs on an individual basis.

If at all possible, ask for a room close to the elevator, or a manned station on each floor. It is extremely important that there is an emergency button in the room, easy to activate, in the bathroom too, if possible.

Check if the facility has available services such as: nursing services, at least for most of the day, a house doctor with visiting hours during the week, and banking services available close by. Are there post office services available? Is there a social worker? Is there security 24 hours a day? Does the facility provide the residents with laundry services?

Some of the assisted living facilities provide a full meal plan; some provide small kitchenettes and only a partial meal plan. If it is the latter, make sure there is a place to purchase food nearby. If you are in a place that provides a full meal plan, check if they can accommodate special needs, such as diabetic diet, low-salt diet, kosher diet, etc.

You may want to pay for two weeks or a month as a trial period, before you commit to a situation which is basically for the rest of your life.   It is advisable to do so before selling one's belonging and/or giving up one's home and most of its contents.

I have met people who were very surprised by how much the arrangement suited them, socially and physically. On the other hand, I know people who were happy that they had not sold their homes, and given away their belongings, because they found assisted living restrictive. It is advisable to check out a few assisted living facilities, even if the first one looks great just to make sure that it is the *one*. Each of the facilities vary by services, size of room and grounds, type of population, activities, number of support staff, and other factors.

It is wise to compare the cost of services among different facilities. Assisted living facilities provide a similar range of services, but the costs may vary considerably.

The following is a guideline for you to help compare costs and ask the right questions when assessing each facility:

Entrance and initial assessment fee: $_____

Selected unit and basic service package fee: $_____

Meals: $_____

Housekeeping: $_____

Personal laundry or linen services: $_____

Medication management or assistance: $_____

Personal care assistance
(Bathing, dressing, eating): $_____

Recreational activities: $_____

Transportation: $_____

Telephone service: $_____

Cable television: $_____

Beauty shop: $_____

Other charges: $_____

Total monthly charges: $_____

Another factor to check out is the staff of the facility. There should be enough personnel to provide all the services and maintain the facility as a safe environment for its residents. There should be a nurse on the premises 24/7.

A frequently asked question is: Which is better, a larger facility or a smaller facility? There is no precise answer to this question. Small facilities provide more personal attention and a more home-like feeling, yet a larger facility is likely to offer a wider selection of services.

In a large facility you may lose some of the personal feeling, and you may have a hard time remembering the names of many people, but there will be a greater range of activities, sports - such as golf, tennis, maybe a pool with a swimming program) as well as social activities like parties, dances, sing-along sessions.

The decision should be based on personal priorities. If you feel better in smaller surroundings, and it is important to you to know the people with whom you share the facility, a small assisted living facility may work better for you.

More outgoing elderly might like a wide variety of social events, social contacts, and a mixed society, which includes the society outside the residential facility. This cannot be provided by small assisted living facilities.

When buying a house, you tend to check and recheck all factors on which you would base your decision, such as the neighborhood, safety, shopping areas, transportation proximity, and rate of availability. Look for the same when you evaluate an assisted living facility. The only element you do not have to be concerned with is the school system.

As with purchasing a house, keep coming back, evaluating and reevaluating until you are sure that this is the right place for you.

The cost of living in an assisted living facility varies from facility to facility, from city to city, and from state to state. It also varies by the different levels of luxury that the facilities offer. When researching costs for the assisted living options, we found such a wide range that it is almost impossible to generalize. Not only did the basic fees differ, but added fees for services were also varied widely.

The prices below were collected from calls across the country to many assisted living facilities offering as little as just small apartment units to luxuries and large units. Some of the facilities have a full range of services, such as 3 meals a day, all housekeeping chores, nurse on the premises, etc.

The facilities we contacted varied in size, some as small as 4 to 8 residential units, others as large as 260 units. At some of the facilities, the residents rent the unit; in others, the unit is purchased.

If you consider buying, you should beware of all the restrictions that can come into play if you want to sell the unit later. If there are restrictions that will make it difficult to sell the unit, if there is a need to have the approval of the potential buyer by management or a residents' committee, or if there is a fee that you need to pay to the management company, you may want to opt for rental rather than purchase.

Here some of the prices to give you an idea:

The lowest-price assisted living unit we found in the Northeast included a semi-private room, 3 meals a day, weekly change of linen, and light cleaning. The cost was $1,650 per month (rental). Any additional services, such as medication reminders, or assistance with bathing or dressing, would be charged separately, either by hourly fee ($19 per hour), or per service. That particular facility required a 12 month lease agreement.

Sixty five percent of the facilities that we polled quoted the monthly cost between $2,800 and $4,800 per month. This represents the basic cost of renting a residential unit, which is sometimes a one bedroom and other times just a studio. This includes housekeeping, meals, recreational facilities, and activities. Some places have an entry fee - commonly between $5,000 and $10,000 - which is nonrefundable.

Many facilities have levels of services added to the basic cost. If a resident requires assistance with bathing, with administering medication, and transportation, it will add to his or her monthly cost. Most services will have one, two or three levels of service, adding between $300 and $900 per level to the monthly cost. Extra services may be charged by the hour, and the cost can run between $12 and $30 per hour.

A few of the facilities quoted per-day rates with a one-year contract. One facility's daily fee of $175 covers the cost of a one-bedroom unit, all meals, and recreational facilities, such as tennis, pool, and a golf course. The annual cost of $63,875 includes light housekeeping, linen change, and clean towels, but the resident is responsible for personal laundry. Any additional services are the resident's responsibility.

Very few of the assisted living facilities that we called offered their units for purchase - most were rentals. But like retirement communities, the units that were for sale were priced as low as $120,000, and as high as $457,000.

As with every option, one should well research the place that is of interest to them, and compare prices with other assisted living facilities in the area. When you find a facility that you think will be suitable for you or for your parent, work out an arrangement with the management where you can try the facility for a month to make sure that it is indeed the right choice.

SHARED HOUSING

This option allows people to share their housing situation with non-family members. Sharing a household with one or two people will split the cost, share chores, and decrease loneliness. If the home is shared with another person in fairly the same situation, with similar needs, it may be a successful match. This arrangement can be used with younger people as well as older, like students or working people that need to live in the area.

The shared housing set-up may allow people who live alone in their apartment or private house, to remain in their home as they age. At times the cost of staying home becomes a burden and a drain on their resources. Some will sell their home and seek another option; others will do everything possible to remain in their home. Their home is more to them than a living space, it is their past, possibly the place in which they raised their children, and it is their place of comfort. They may have lived there for many years, and they do not want to change their living arrangement.

The shared housing arrangement should be carefully evaluated. You should make sure that each person has privacy. You have to be willing to provide closet space, maybe an extra bathroom if available, or make space available in a bathroom you will share.

For this arrangement to work, all has to be shared: utility expenses, monthly cost of mortgage, maintenance, etc. Some people choose to keep food expenses separate, but there is always a worry that the other person will eat "my" food. So the best scenario would be to share food expenses too.

You should meet the person who will possibly share the household with you or your loved one at least a few times to find out as much as possible about them. A background check should be made. A similar culture, age, and background would best promote compatibility.

In many cases, the partnership to share a household stems from friendships or family relations- people who have known one another for many years, enjoy each other's company, and trust one another. If the person is unknown to you, the selection process should be much more intense and careful; after all you'll be letting a stranger into the house.

Medical history should also be taken into account. You do not want to share a household with someone who requires a great deal of care. But keep in mind that, after years of living together, health needs can change.

The success of a shared household depends on many components, and if any one of them is removed, the whole arrangement may fail. The following could negatively affect the arrangement:

1. Financial changes that could cause one of the partners to default financially. Financial unbalance will cause the arrangement to end.

2. If personal conflict occurs, it may cause the arrangement to end.

3. If a member decides to leave, due to health, financial reasons, or any other reason, a new household member must be sought, if the unit is to be maintained.

4. Serious illness of one partner may cause great hardship on others. Considering the age of the partners in the shared household, this is quite likely.

All of these points must be taken into account when considering a shared household for you or your parent. This option is a good one, but it is not for everyone.

The shared household option will, in my opinion, become more popular, partly because the baby boomers are more equipped to maintain their independence for many years and are financially better off. Due to significant cost increases, sharing expenses makes sense. While this option provides the elderly with independent living, he or she may use many of the support services the community provides, such as senior centers, transportation, etc.

Go to www.eldercohousing.org for more information, as well as our Internet site www.goldernyearsgolder.com.

RETIREMENT COMMUNITIES

Retirement communities have become very popular. Many people switch from owning their own homes, in a community at large, to living in retirement communities when they are in their fifties or sixties. Some middle-aged people are purchasing units in retirement communities before they actually retire. In many areas throughout the country, this type of investment turned out to be a good one. If we want to generalize, ten years ago the same unit would have cost about 50 percent less than it would today.

These communities are basically individual units, most often one floor that consists of one or two bedrooms, and are built to be very functional and suited to aging people. Most of the retirement communities include a pool, tennis courts, social club, and gym. In the upper-end communities there may be a golf club and health clinic along with a local doctor.

The prices for these units differ from community to community and from state to state, and it totally depends on the local real estate market. When choosing this option, you should consider the cost, not only of the unit at the time of purchase, but also the monthly maintenance fee. The questions to ask: Will the maintenance cover all outdoor services, including the maintenance of the outside of the unit, such as upkeep of the roof, exterior walls, and sidewalk?

When you tour retirement communities, examine the interior to determine how well it will accommodate your needs in the future, when you may not ambulate as well as you do now. Are the doors wide so a wheelchair can fit through them? Can the bathroom accommodate wheelchairs and walkers? Are there safety bars in the bathroom, or can they be installed? Does the entrance to your unit have too many steps? Can a ramp be made, or is there some restriction on that? Many communities do not like any exterior changes, so the uniformity of the community's look stays consistent.

If you like the community you are visiting and the price is within your range, make sure you visit a few times at different times of the day, as well as on the weekend. This will give you a picture of what kind of community it is, and how the people interact. Look at the evening activities and how residents are encouraged to participate.

Look at the safety procedures. Is there a system for emergencies in place? Is there night coverage for crises? Is it easy to shop for necessities or does one need a car for all shopping? Is public transportation available?

In most cases, prices can be negotiated. Check if special rates for mortgages are available for the elderly in your state. Some banks also provide special rates for the elderly with special guarantees.

When researching the cost and availability of retirement communities, we discovered that they are popping up all over America. Builders, who just few years ago were building rows of houses for the average American family, have begun building specifically for the retiring population.

As in every industry in this country, builders are beginning to realize that the baby boomers are coming into the senior sector of the American population. Specializing in building for seniors has become a very lucrative business.

With retirement communities being built all over, it is understandable that the range of prices is quite varied. One can find two- bedroom units for as little as $45,000, with a reasonable monthly maintenance fee of $270 in smaller towns throughout the United States.

The more luxurious retirement communities quoted prices in the range of $550,000 to a million dollars. So it is no surprise that the monthly maintenance cost is also very high, hovering between $1,800 and $3,000.

Some of the more luxurious communities offer one or two pools, first class golf courses, tennis courts, libraries, gathering halls, and daily activities, such as yoga, exercise classes, art, and continuing education programs affiliated with local colleges.

When you choose the retirement community you want to become your home, or the home of your loved one, you should first consider if the price per unit and monthly payments are right for your budget.

The second thing that you should determine is if the community offers what you are looking for. If you like to sit on your patio and read, or watch sports on your television, you may not want to pay for the tennis courts or the golf courses if you won't use them.

Communities that offer fewer recreational activities tend to be less costly in purchase price, as well as in monthly maintenance fees.

As with any other large purchase, you should get the conditions and restrictions for future sale of the unit or for leaving the unit to your heirs in writing. You want to make sure that there are no unexpected preconditions that can complicate a sale of the unit or a transfer.

RESIDENTIAL CARE FACILITIES

Residential care facilities basically provide monthly rental of a room, with minimal oversight, and usually do not even have a nurse. Some of the very basic facilities cost as little as the monthly Social Security income the person receives. Others can cost a few thousand dollars per month.

Almost all residents of such a facility are highly functional individuals, and are mostly left to themselves. At the lower end, these facilities are very simple. Some can be quite depressing, and they house a lot of people who may suffer from mental illnesses to various degrees.

In New York during the 1980s, many mental institutions released a number of patients of moderate levels of illness, who were expected to be easily absorbed into the community. It did not work exactly, as many ended up in the street. But some did find homes - many came to live in residential facilities which were basically room and board places. All it required to open one was a relatively easy to get C license and the ability to fill the beds. A nurse was brought in to administer medication. Some of these places looked worse than the institutions the residents came from.

Most of these places did nothing at the time to provide residents with any activities, leaving them bored and unmotivated. Some were heavily medicated and totally removed from human contact and stimulation. In some places, social services were required and a visiting social worker would show up once or twice per week.

In many cases people who worked for this type of business had no or very minimal experience in the health field. For most residential care facilities, the basic deal was to make a profit; they provided very poorly for the residents, who were either lonely or mentally impaired, with no one to stand up for them.

With time, the residential care facilities became much more opulent and filled with high-end residents. The rooms were decorated to appeal to middle- and upper-class residents. The range of services also increased. Most have a nurse on the premises and a visiting doctor and social worker. The menu also improved with time as residents became more demanding.

Cost can still be based on Social Security income plus pension or an added monthly fee. But some places, such as New York City, the expense can run as high as $5,500 per month. This monthly cost does not include a meal plan, which can run from $30 to $75 per day.

Residential facilities, as well as retirement communities, are not covered by Medicaid or Medicare. Some long-term insurance plans will cover residential care facilities, or partial care in retirement communities. You should very carefully read the small print in your long-term care contract.

LONG-TERM FACILITIES

NURSING HOMES

As more options have become available for the elderly and the ill, fewer choose the nursing home option. Still, some 1.5 million Americans are currently residing in nursing homes across the United States. This represents a small segment of the 65 year and older population, but as the numbers of this aging population grow, the numbers of nursing home residents will increase as well.

Nursing homes in all states are licensed, regulated, and/or certified by different agencies within the given state. In most cases, the health department of the state will be the one to do the regulating and licensing. In some states it may be under the Department of Health, or the Health Care Financing Administration. The agencies and departments doing the regulations and inspections may vary from state to state; go under different titles, and/or overlap. The final say in most cases is given to the Department of Health.

Many of the elderly and their family members find nursing homes less desirable than assisted living facilities and residential care situations. They feel nursing homes rob the elderly of their independence, signaling mental and physical decline, and will most likely be the place they will live out the end of their lives.

Nonetheless, for many elderly people, a nursing home may be a good choice or the only choice available. Many doctors will recommend a nursing home for recovery stay after a stroke or bad bone fracture. The patients can receive rehabilitative services, after which many of them can return to their permanent residences. This type of care is often referred to as temporary rehabilitation, skilled nursing, and transitional care.

Most people who enter nursing homes do so in need of full medical care for conditions from which they will not recover. Other problems that bring people to nursing homes are incontinence, memory disorders, mental disorders, strokes, ambulation problems, terminal and chronic illnesses, or the loss of caregivers.

The single most important reason for a person to go into a nursing home is if they need care at a level that they may not be able to receive at home or in any other living situation, such as assisted living.

Nursing homes are called many different names: nursing centers, care centers, skilled nursing centers, convalescent center and chronic illness centers. Most provide full range of skilled nursing and medical services; some also provide rehabilitation and occupational therapy.

These long-term facilities provide a wide range of services from assistance with bathing, dressing, feeding, transferring in and out of bed, and toileting. Most residents in nursing homes are either mentally or physically impaired. According to statistical data, 40% of all Americans

65 years and over will spend some time in their life in a nursing home or rehabilitation center. Of all the people who enter nursing homes, more than half of them will remain there for the remainder of their lives.

The nursing home industry is currently highly regulated, but it would still be wise to research the facility you are considering for any violations. As for sources of payments that are available, Medicare will not pay for nursing home care, unless it is rehabilitative care for a condition from which one will recover. Most of these conditions are strokes and fractures. Medicaid will provide funding for lower income patients. To qualify for Medicaid funding, documentation is needed to show financial status and need. A paper trail of financial history, going back three years, is required to qualify for Medicaid. Any financial changes your parents want to make, such as transferring some of their assets, would best be done five years before needing a nursing home. So the earlier you plan for such eventuality, the better.

Long term facilities may also provide a varied list of services, among them physical therapy, skin care, respiratory care, tube feeding, etc. Skilled care is state regulated, and may vary from state to state. Each state has specific offices that deal with information on nursing homes in general as well as specific nursing homes.

Nursing homes usually have two or three levels of care, ranging from that which is appropriated for highly active people who participate in all social and recreational activities to totally care-dependent residents. You will find that the higher the floor, the more care is required for the residents, who are less independent, responsive, and interactive.

When touring nursing homes for your loved one make sure that you visit the upper floors, check for urine odors and residents wandering aimlessly, and take note of residents' personal hygiene. Check also for "storaging" of confused residents seated in geriatric chairs in dining rooms and recreational rooms for long periods of time. Those floors are usually not included in the tours given to potential residents and their families. It is also important to find out the ratio of workers to residents in any given facility.

It may be wise to seek out a not-for-profit facility, which tend to pay their workers slightly higher salaries, thus they tend to be happier with their work. Nursing homes that have been around for a long time tend to be better established, and have a track record that can be checked.

There are state regulations as to the ratio of workers to residents, number of baths per week the residents are to be provided with, as well as how many feeders work in a given facility. These numbers should be checked for all shifts, day and night.

These numbers are very important, as they directly relate to the quality of care provided to your loved one. If there are not enough feeders, say, it will suggest that some people in need of feeding are rushed through meals. If a worker's time spent feeding a patient is limited the patient will most likely not receive adequate nutrition.

Strike up a conversation with some workers, try to get a sense if they are forthcoming and friendly; this is what you want for your loved one. Observe the interaction between nurses, nurse's aides, and the patient. Is there a great deal of vocal stimulation? Is the patient engaged by the staff? Do the patients interact with each other? All of this is very important; this will be the daily life of your loved one's daily routine. Be prepared to spend one or two hours on such a visit, or even more. It is not a bad idea to visit a few times, at different times of the day, or maybe during a weekend.

During such visits you should watch for the personal cleanliness of the residents, their rooms, and the general pleasantness of the environment. Ask to speak to family members of residents that live in the particular nursing home; if the administrators refuse, seek out another nursing home.

Demands for nursing home services are lessening. There are a few reasons for this: one, the realization that the quality of life in them leaves something to be desired and problems in nursing homes have been highlighted in the media; and two, the availability of other options.

One should be aware of the fact that more than 75% of nursing home residents become impoverished in one year. One should consider long-term insurance that will protect against depleting one's assets in a very short time. Long-term insurance should be looked at many years before the needs accrue; the cost of such insurance will then be lowest. See the chapter on Long Term Insurance in this book.

For seniors in need of nursing home care, but who may not want the traditional nursing home, the Green House Project, whose website is www.thegreenhouseproject.com, may be of interest to them. This organization develops small group homes that offer medical services in a much friendlier and more personal environment than the traditional facilities.

The cost of a nursing home varies greatly, from city to city, state to state. Many factors come into play when cost for nursing home is set. It depends on location, size, services offered, and demand of the given facility. Some nursing homes have waiting lists; some are forever doing marketing to try to fill their beds. When evaluating a nursing home and looking at the price tag, you should understand how the price is set, and why it's so different from one nursing home to another.

So how do you go about finding a nursing home? Although some people find them through the Yellow Pages, most of us prefer to find a nursing home through recommendations. One of the sources of recommendation is the local hospital. Every hospital has a Social Services department that can provide recommendations for nursing homes in the area. The social workers are likely to explain the differences among them, and they will also know if the specific nursing home is suitable for your needs.

Other sources of referral may be your doctor, family members, friends, and people who have experience with finding a nursing home for their loved one. Consult the Nursing Home Association of your state for recommendations in finding nursing home facilities. You can find your state's Nursing Home Association on our site: www.goldenyearsgolden.com.

It is not an easy task to find the right nursing home. What one needs most when evaluating a nursing home is time. You should not be rushed, though in reality we do not always have the luxury of time.

When you find a nursing home that you like, you can request that your parent stay for a month in the facility, so they can see how they like it. During that month you do not have to make any commitments nor do you have to sell their home. This way there is always a way to back out if they are unhappy in the nursing home. Also if you let them make the decision, they will still feel in control of their life and will be partners in the decision-making.

Some of the nursing homes are very beautifully decorated and include quality furniture. Patients' rooms look like a room in your home, and some nursing homes will allow the patient to bring their own furniture especially if they are staying in a single room. This type of nursing home tends to be higher priced.

But most nursing homes look more institutional with less homely décor, making it sometime difficult for a patient to differentiate his or her room from another room. Science has been clear about the need for visual stimulation to the elderly, the sick, and the lonely. If every room, corridor, dining room, and recreation room is gray and cold, it promotes depression, indifference, and isolation. There is no question that you should stay away from that kind of nursing home, even if other factors are suitable for your parent, such as cost and distance to your home.

Another issue to look at is the number of complaints, if any, that have been brought against a specific nursing home. This can be checked through your local Office of the Aged, or your state health department. Contact the State Survey Agency in your state, or the state in which the nursing home is located, if it is different. The State Survey Agency can tell you if the given nursing home is licensed and/or certified, and if there are any legal actions that have been taken against it. There are other governmental offices you can use for information, but this a good place to start.

When you are looking for a nursing home for your mother or father, it goes without saying that you want them to be in the best nursing home possible. To make sure that a particular nursing home is the right place, you need to do some research. First, you need to visit more than one or two nursing homes. Compare sizes, and number of services offered, such as physical therapy and rehabilitation.

Extended medical staff availability should be considered, as well as if support equipment is available and is in good condition. Does the nursing home have a night staff sufficient to handle emergencies? Some nursing homes have limited staffing on night shifts, which can be outright dangerous in case of an emergency, such as a fire.

You may want to see an activity calendar, a month or two back, to see the types of activities offered, and the number of activities, daily, weekly, and monthly. Ask how residents are encouraged to participate in the activities. Is there residents' council and do they have input in the nursing home life? There should be minutes of their meetings, usually filed with the social worker's office.

Each state's requirements are different. You need to check with your state's health department, regarding what services, such as how many times a patient is bathed in a week, are required by the state. How many workers are required for a 30 patient unit? How many feeders are required to be on hand? Are the hallways wide enough to accommodate wheelchairs? Some of the old nursing homes have narrow doorways and narrow hallways, making it difficult to maneuver through them.

In your visits to assess potential nursing homes for your loved one, you should check if privacy in patients' rooms is respected, and if their belongings are protected in their room. Can they have their own telephone installed in their room? All these things add up to reflect the quality of everyday life. I have seen nursing homes in which residents wandered in and out of other residents' rooms, taking personal items of others. Ask the representative of the nursing home you are visiting how they discourage that kind of practice.

The sources of payment for a nursing home are as follows:

a. Personal: you pay out of pocket. You may use savings, investments, and assets you receive upon the sale of your house.

b. Medicaid. This is a joint federal and state program that will pay for health and long-term custodial care for Americans with low income and no other resources. Medicaid recipients are required to pay a share of cost from their income toward the nursing home cost upon entering.

c. Long-term insurance: Whether your policy will provide coverage for nursing home services, partially or fully, depends on the policy you have. You should check when purchasing such a policy, what the requirements to activate the policy are, and who ultimately makes the decision that it is time to enter a nursing home; i.e., the senior's personal physician or the insurer's doctors. You can see that the latter may leave you or your parent at the mercy of the insurance company. At times the insurance will have a bridge time, where the policy kicks in after the first, second or third month. You should know that at time of purchase to avoid surprises.

d. Medicare will cover short stays, under certain conditions, mostly for rehabilitative services.

There are many different checklists to use, but use what works best for you. Following is a checklist to use as a guideline:

NURSING HOME CHECKLIST

Name of Nursing Home:_____

Date of Visit:_____

Yes / No

Basic Information
The nursing home is Medicare-certified.   **YES/ NO**

The nursing home is Medicaid-certified.   **YES/ NO**

The nursing home has the level of care needed
(e.g., skilled, custodial); has a bed available.   **YES/ NO**

The nursing home has special services if needed
in a separate unit (e.g., dementia, ventilator,
or rehabilitation), and has a bed available.   **YES/ NO**

The nursing home is located close enough
for friends and family to visit.   **YES/ NO**

Resident Appearance
Residents are clean, appropriately dressed for
the season or time of day, and well groomed.   **YES/ NO**

Nursing Home Living Spaces
The nursing home is free of unpleasant odors,
and appears to be clean and well-kept.   **YES/ NO**

The temperature in the nursing home is
comfortable for residents.   **YES/ NO**

There is good lighting throughout   **YES/ NO**

Noise levels in the dining room and other
common areas are comfortable.   **YES/ NO**

Smoking is not allowed or restricted to certain areas
of the nursing home.   **YES/ NO**

Furnishings are sturdy, yet comfortable and
attractive and are placed in a way that
promotes safety.   **YES/ NO**

Staff
The relationship between the staff and the residents
appears to be warm, polite, and respectful.   **YES/ NO**

All staff members wear name tags.   **YES/ NO**

Staff is respectful of residents (e.g., they knock
on the door before entering a resident's room
and refer to residents by name)   **YES/NO**

The nursing home offers a training and
continuing education program for all staff, and
staff receives annual medical checkups.   **YES/ NO**

The nursing home does background checks on
all staff.   **YES/ NO**

The guide on your tour knows the residents by
name and is recognized by them.   **YES/ NO**

There is a full-time registered nurse (RN) in the
nursing home at all times, other than the
administrator.   **YES/ NO**

The same team of nurses and certified nursing
assistants (CNAs) work with the same resident
4 to 5 days per week.   **YES/ NO**

CNAs work with a reasonable number of residents.	**YES/ NO**
CNAs are involved in care-planning meetings.	**YES/ NO**
There is a full-time social worker on staff.	**YES/ NO**
There is a licensed doctor on staff. Is he or she there daily? Can he or she be reached at all times?	**YES/ NO**
The nursing home's management team has worked together for at least one year.	**YES/ NO**

Residents' Rooms

Residents may have personal belongings and/or furniture in their rooms.	**YES/ NO**
Each resident has storage space (closet and drawers) in his or her room.	**YES/ NO**
Each resident has a window in his or her bedroom.	**YES/ NO**
Residents have access to a personal telephone and television.	**YES/ NO**
Residents have a choice of roommates.	**YES/ NO**
Water pitchers are available in residents' rooms.	**YES/NO**
There are policies and procedures to protect residents' possessions.	**YES/ NO**

Hallways, Stairs, Lounges, and Bathrooms

Exits are clearly marked.	**YES/ NO**
There are quiet common areas where residents can visit with friends and family.	**YES/ NO**

The nursing home has smoke detectors and
sprinklers.   **YES/ NO**

All common areas, resident rooms, and
doorways are designed for wheelchair use.   **YES/ NO**

There are handrails in the hallways and grab bars
in the bathrooms.   **YES/ NO**

Menus and Food
Residents have a choice of food items at each meal.
(Ask if your favorite foods are served.)   **YES/ NO**

Nutritious snacks are available upon request.   **YES/ NO**

Staff help residents eat and drink at
mealtimes if help is needed.   **YES/ NO**

Activities
Residents, including those who are unable to
leave their rooms, may choose to take part in a
variety of activities.   **YES/ NO**

The nursing home has outdoor areas for resident
use and staff help residents go outside.   **YES/ NO**

The nursing home has an active volunteer program.   **YES/NO**

Religious services are available for different religions. **YES/NO**

Safety and Care
The nursing home has an emergency evacuation
plan and holds regular fire drills.   **YES/ NO**

Residents get preventative care, like an annual flu
shot, to help them remain healthy.   **YES/ NO**

Residents may still see their personal doctors,
if they so choose. **YES/ NO**

The nursing home has an arrangement with
a nearby hospital for emergencies. **YES/ NO**

Care plan meetings are held at times that are
convenient for residents and family members
to attend whenever possible. **YES/ NO**

The nursing home has corrected all deficiencies
(failure to meet one or more Federal or State
requirements) on its last state inspection report. **YES/ NO**

The cost for a resident in a nursing home can range widely. Not only do the prices vary among different nursing homes from state to state, but within a state the prices can vary significantly.

We randomly called several nursing homes, and skilled nursing home facilities, including small nursing homes with no more than 20 beds that specialize in specific needs, and facilities that have 350 or 400 beds.

We looked at costs for private rooms and semi-private rooms. Private rooms increase the cost for the resident by between 10 to 20 percent on average.

The costs quoted to us by the nursing homes basically covered bed and board, and reflected the charge for a semi-private room. Although, all nursing homes we spoke to have nurses on their staff, specific residents needs, such as medication and physical therapy, are individually billed to the resident's account. All linens, towels, and laundry costs are included, but personal clothing is again the responsibility of the resident.

We found that nursing home costs are significantly higher in the Northeast, as well as on the West Coast, with patches of the Midwest representing the lower span of the nursing home cost. In general, the annual cost for a semi-private nursing home stay ranges from $32,000 to $142,000. Of course, we did not call all of the thousands of nursing homes throughout the country, but this is a good sampling. These amounts reflect the ballpark figures for private costs. If you or your parent are lucky enough to have long-term insurance that will totally or partially cover the nursing home cost, or if you qualify for Medicaid, you do not have to worry about the cost. All you need is to find a facility that will serve you best.

Just a reminder, when researching different nursing homes, make sure to have in writing what the price covers, so there are no surprise expenses each month.

Contact information regarding nursing homes in your state can be found on our site: www.goldenyearsgolden.com .

Case # 6

Many years ago, as a student, I worked part-time in a nursing home. It was the first time in my life that I had been in an environment that cared for the elderly, and seniors were at different levels of functioning. Many were fully alert and highly functioning. I grew up without relatives who were elderly. Both sets of my grandparents died in the Holocaust, so I did not have the exposure to elderly people. I found them fascinating; each could be my grandmother or grandfather. Thus began my interest and love for the field of geriatrics.

One of the residents was a very quiet lady that kept a great deal to herself, and refused most invitations to activities, caught my attention. At times I saw her in the library, turning pages absent-mindedly. But mostly I found it fascinating to watch her sitting outdoors, weather permitting, bundled up, eyes closed, sunbathing her face. She always looked so peaceful, so detached from the world around her. The staff told me that she had been doing this for years, a few hours at a time.

Slowly, I developed a friendly relationship with her. It took a long time for her to open up, but finally she seemed to enjoy spending time with me. She talked to me about her life, about her kids, their lives, her late husband. But what I wanted to know was why she sat for hours with her eyes closed. I finally asked. "Remembering," she said. "Remembering?" I asked.

She had a whole theory about it; when you're young; you're too busy to experience everything. You fall in love, marry, give life to children, watch them grow, watch them become strong adults, navigate through life. And then, joyously, you see your kids establish their own families. How wonderful, how fulfilling, the pride a parent feels, the joy.

After the kids are on their own, and they do not require all your attention anymore, you renew your acquaintance with the man you married, before the rest of them stepped into your life. You again discover the very things that made your heart beat faster - the smile and the tender touch. You rediscover the "us," that somehow got lost over the years, and it is so wonderful to find it again.

"So we started to travel again, just the two of us, feeling young again. Discovering ourselves, as well as rediscovering the world. It was wonderful, both retired, we saved enough to be secure in our old age, and could enjoy the traveling without worrying about the cost", she told me.

"We finally traveled to Alaska, and China, both childhood dreams, as well as Africa, and Israel, and threw in a few cruises for good measure. All were wonderful trips, building memories for future years. And it lasted through our seventies and into our mid eighties. And it all felt like being in our thirties, or at the most our forties."

Then the husband had a stroke, and within three days he was gone. A partner, a soul mate, was gone in three days. Within two months of laying her husband to rest, she sold their home, splitting everything between the kids. They were supportive and loving, but she did not want to be a burden to them, so she picked a nursing home with their help (those were pre-residential care or assisted living facility times). This nursing home looked good, and the best part was that it was near her daughter, so here she was.

So now she sits down, she explained, and quietly lets the sun dance on her face while she brings back all the memories, each one, joyously remembered, and cherished. The weddings, the births, the holiday celebrations, the trips, all remembered with so much love.

I was so touched by what she told me. I thanked her for sharing all that with me, and I could understand her looking back, enjoying it. But nonetheless I thought, she should be more involved in today, in the now. So we started a personal history group. The group would meet and share past experiences. And she became very active in this group. As its leader, her life took a turn, bringing out the social person that she was. The program was in high demand so we ran it a few times a week, and the other residents just loved it, each bringing into it their own cherished memories. The program was called "The Memory Album."

Through the years, whenever the opportunity has presented itself, I told the seniors, whether individuals in home care or groups in long-term facilities, of the wonderful activity: the Memory Album. I always found that people responded to it happily and benefited from it greatly, for the mental stimulation it provided, and the joy it brought.

I, too, now collect memories for my album.

REHABILITATIVE CARE CENTERS

Short-Term Facilities

Those types of facilities were developed more and more by nursing homes for the income they generate and are for short-term stays. They provide services for recovery for patients after surgery, fractures, strokes, etc.

Most rehabilitation centers consist of a designated number of beds in hospitals and skilled nursing homes, although there are also fully separate rehabilitation facilities. Whatever form they are in, short-term facilities usually provide physical therapy, speech therapy, occupational therapy, as well as IV therapy, monitored by an RN, tube feeding, sterile dressing for bed sores and post-surgery wounds care.

Medicare will pay (as per the Medicare Handbook) 100 days of rehabilitation, but in reality your parent will need to spend three consecutive nights in hospital to qualify for rehabilitation. Your parent will also need skilled care related to the condition for which they were treated in the hospital; it also has to be a condition from which they are expected to recover in a reasonable amount of time.

One can only receive rehabilitation services from a Medicare-certified facility within 30 days of being discharged from a hospital. The doctor must certify that the patient needs rehabilitation or skilled nursing care for Medicare to pay for it.

If you or your parent qualifies and meet those guidelines, Medicare will pay for a limited period of time. The first 20 days of rehabilitation are covered 100% by Medicare. After 20 days, Medicare will pay all costs of rehabilitation, after the co-pay, which the patient pays. In 2007, the co-pay was $119, and is adjusted annually. Medigap and Medicaid will cover the co-pay – (Medicaid depends on the financial status of the patient). After 100 days, Medicare stops paying. If the patient does not qualify for Medicaid and has no supplementary insurance, private funds may have to be used.

Due to the fact that this type of facility is meant for short-term use, most people go to the rehabilitative facility that the doctor or hospital recommends. This choice does not require much evaluation on your part. All the facility has to offer is the proper rehabilitative services that you or your parent may need.

SPECIAL CARE UNIT

Special care units are facilities dealing with special needs, such as Alzheimer's, other type of dementia, or respiratory care, etc. Such units are usually attached to nursing homes, care centers, or chronic hospitals.

With all the new options out there, the old nursing home option is not the only one, and people do not need to rush to consider that option. So the nursing homes are trying to develop special units and be more attractive to potential residents and their families.

If you research the market, you will find nursing homes that have designated one or more floors to be for provision of specialized care. There are units for respiratory treatments, there are units specializing in Alzheimer's and other dementia care. There are also units for rehabilitation, to which patients with injuries are transferred directly from hospitals for physical rehabilitation.

This fairly new development provides for increased income to the nursing home, and the specialized care is covered by most insurance and best of all by Medicare.

If your loved one has been hospitalized due to some injury or trauma, and you are informed by the medical staff that he or she will require rehabilitative services, ask them which facilities they work with and recommend.

It is smart to make a trip to the facility and compare it with others. And most importantly, check if they are known for quality services in the particular type of injury that your loved one suffered. You can check this with the doctor and with the social services of the hospital.

Check in the Medicare section for the coverage of rehabilitation therapy days, and the specific qualifications needed in your case.

It is important to explain to your loved one that you are not putting them in a nursing home, and their stay in the facility is temporary and only for rehabilitation.

Some hospitals also have rehabilitation departments, and will transfer the patient to their own unit. But you should check for quality and area of specialization there too. It is in within your right to request another rehabilitation center which you know to be better, but be sure to check that it qualifies for Medicare, so you don't have to foot the bill.

HOSPICE CARE

Hospice services are provided to patients with end-stage illnesses. Initially, hospice services were provided to patients with cancer in their homes. But in the last 10 to 15 years, hospice service has become available in most hospitals, long-term institutions, as well as in residential care facilities. Medicare and Medicaid, as well as most insurance plans, provide hospice care coverage. Medicare and Medicaid require prescriptions from the patient's doctor stating that the patient has six months or less to live. After that period, if the patient needs more hospice care, re-qualifying will be required of the patient. Health insurance coverage varies from one company to another and it is prudent to check what is included, what is not, and all the prerequisites.

Now Hospice services cover not only patients with cancer, but also those with Alzheimer's, cardiac disease, renal failure, and any debilitating illnesses at the terminal stage.

Medicare hospice coverage will provide an interdisciplinary team, skilled in pain management, symptom control, and bereavement assistance. In addition, it will pay for durable medical equipment, such as oxygen equipment, walkers and wheelchairs, as well as medications to control pain that was ordered by the hospice team.

Most hospice services will include family members or friends of the patient who provide support and guidance throughout the months of struggle with the illness, helping them with pain and the acceptance process.

Hospice services can be recommended to you by a family doctor, nursing home, home care agency, or the office of information at every hospital in your neighborhood. Hospice services can be provided even if home care services are also being given. The aide will provide the care under the direction of the hospice service team.

Some hospice services can be set up with a religious affiliation, so if it is appropriate to your loved one, it may bring comfort to them in the last months of their life.

The life end services of the hospices are provided as per need, and with the level of acceptance of the person who is ill. They vary from patient to patient, regardless of whether they are provided in the patient's home, the hospital, or a nursing home, etc. For hospice contact information in your state, go to our site www.goldenyearsgolden.com .

Case # 7

A very good friend of mine, a woman in her 50s was diagnosed with lung cancer. She had been a smoker for many years, but in the last ten years, she slowly reduced her smoking, until she finally stopped altogether.

Ever the optimist, she immersed herself into researching the field regarding disease immediately after the diagnosis and initial shock – looking into the available therapies, and the prognosis for her type of illness. It was very confusing and she was overwhelmed by the amount of information out there. Having no medical background, it was very difficult for her to sort out the good from the bad as well as the therapies that could apply to her condition and those that were totally unsuitable for her.

Many times we spoke about her disease, and how she was proceeding with the treatment. She followed all new developments in the treatments of her type of cancer. And she never lost her hope and belief that she would beat it. She was so brave.

Three years after the original diagnosis, after numerous up and downs, she was told by her doctors that she was losing the battle with the disease. She took it very hard. After few weeks of depression, crying and soul searching; she decided to live the time that was left to her filling it with love, friendship, her family, and the settling of her affairs.

After taking care of her finances, putting a will and a health proxy in place, writing down all the instructions for her kids on what to with her home, and all her possessions, she bravely turned to live the rest of her life, spending as much time with family and friends as possible.

She dealt directly with her doctors, and did not want any information kept from her in an effort to protect her. She asked her doctors to try new therapies on her, for the hope that something would work, and postpone the inevitable. But unfortunately nothing helped.

As her condition worsened and she required more and more help with her daily routines, her doctors offered her to come to the hospital, where her pain could be controlled, and she would be kept pain free as much as possible. She refused, choosing to stay in her own home, in her own bed, with the people and things she loved surrounding her.

That is when the hospice services stepped in. Initially the hospice services provided her with medications for pain control, and some medical supplies that she needed. Later on they provided her with nursing visits, psychological support, a pain management regimen, and all needs that related to her illness.

My friend knew of the grave situation she was in, and she was grateful to the hospice services that made her last weeks bearable; her family too was grateful to the nurses and the aides who came every day to wash her, feed her, and give her the medication she needed to survive another day, with as little pain possible. They were her angels.

Three days before passing away, my friend slipped into a coma. When she died, she looked peaceful. She was surrounded by her family, the nurse and aide from the hospice services agency. They cried together as they said goodbye to this wonderful person.

RESPITE CARE

This type of care can be provided to the elderly and the ill person for short periods of time to elevate the burden of responsibility on the main caregiver. It is geared towards a people who are not able to remain on their own. If such a person is cared for by a family member, a spouse, or a home health aide, for 8, 12, or 24 hours a day, and as the physical and/or mental status changes for the worse, it takes a great deal of emotional and physical toll on the caregiver.

Thus, the need for respite care developed. The care of the patient or elderly person is essentially transferred temporarily to another caregiver.

There are quite a few options out there for respite care, and all you need to do is seek them out. I have found that there are many programs in almost every community that will take in a senior for up to eight hours. The time the elder spends in such a program is the time the main caregiver can rest, and or go about any business they need to take care of.

There are also other possibilities, such as having the senior cared for by a relative or a neighbor. But many seniors do not have a support system - a child, a relative, a friend - that can step in and give a respite to the main caregiver. In the case of the home health aide that is provided through a home care agency, the answer is easy, the agency sends a replacement aide, the care is given, and the permanent caregiver has her or his respite.

Many nursing homes, as well as assisted living facilities and residential care facilities, have programs for short term residential care. If, say, a family who takes care of a parent or grandparent needs to go away for few days or weeks, the elder may be transferred temporarily to a respite care facility. This option leaves the family with no worry for the care and safety of their loved one. This allows the family members and the caregiver an opportunity to recharge, and renew their energy and commitment to the care they are giving.

At the time I was writing this book, the cost for respite care per hour could be found as low as $10 to $12 per hour, or a flat fee of $100 to $130 per 24- hours. Check the program or facility near you that is the best fit for your loved one. It is important that the given program be the right one for them and that it not traumatize them. To decrease the trauma for the senior, you may want to bring him or her to the facility and spend a few hours there with them. This will make them familiar with the place and maybe with some of the staff.

To find such a program check with health facilities in your area.

THE "MY HOUSE" OPTION

Like many people, you may consider the option of bringing your parent or loved one to your house. You'd be surprised how many people decide that the best or the only option is to bring their mother, father, or an elderly relative to live with them.

But as I said before, you need to think very carefully about all implications of such a move. For different reasons, this move may not be a very successful option.

A person moving his or her parent to his home should be commended, but in spite of the desire to make the most and the best of this arrengment, it may not work as well as was hoped.

Consider the following: If in you need to set up a room suitable for your parent in your home, and if it requires one of your children to give up his or her room, it may cause resentment and anger. Routine in your household will have to change, to accommodate an elderly person. Meals will have to be scheduled according to their routine and the elderly tend to eat earlier and retire earlier. It may also require adjusting the menu to provide for whatever restrictions they may have, such as a low-sodium diet, softer food if there are dental problems, etc. The family's dining out routines may be curtailed if the elder is not ambulatory.

Children tend to have a much more active evening, and if my household is an average household in America, dinners are usually served later on in the evening. A great deal of social activities in a household, such as music practice, social visits by friends, television watching, family discussions, and the like, take place in the evening when your parent may not want to be disturbed. The different routines easily can cause friction.

Even if you and your family are willing to adapt to all the changes, it may be much harder for your parent to adjust and accept the change in his or her life. So if it is at all possible, and safe, consider the option of having your parent remain at his or her own home.

If you still think that the best option is for your parent to move in with you, you may want to consider some questions:

Is your house or apartment big enough to accommodate your parent, without causing too much inconvenience to your family? Inconvenience and disruption for a short time is okay, and I am sure that your spouse and kids will all try hard to make the new arrangement work. But long term is a different story, and resentment may build up, and finally explode.

Assess what physical changes you need to make in your house to accommodate your parent, such as safety railings, safety bars in the bathroom, night lights, ramps to the outdoors if needed, etc. Find out how much all the changes will cost beforehand, so you know what you are dealing with. Assess whether your home with all the safety measures put in place is in fact safe for your parent.

Familiarize yourself with your parent's medical situation: What is the care currently required? Can your parent be left alone? How will the illness of your parent progress? Will you be able to handle it down the road, emotionally, physically, and financially?

Make sure to have your family on board with this decision. Make sure to discuss with them, in depth, what is involved in moving your parent to your home. Make sure that you all agree on this decision, or at least accept it, to avoid resentment later on. Do all members of the family understand the sacrifices they will be expected to make?

Although it is very difficult to project and foresee future problems, try hard to do so to make sure that this move will work. If you can predict some of the problems that will or may happen, such as if the illness your parent suffers from brings major changes, such as the need for a wheelchair. If your parent becomes bedridden, can you handle it? I have found that the hardest changes to deal with are the mental changes that may occur in your parent.

If you are employed, will moving your parent to your home impact that? Will you be able to take time off to spend with your parent, at least initially, so your parent can adjust to the new surroundings? If needed, can you take family leave? Is your place of work receptive and understanding to situations such as yours, due to taking your parent to live with you?

Even if not all considerations support such a move, you still may think that this is the only option you have, to move your parent to your home. And it is more than okay, it is admirable, but you should look at the whole picture, and be prepared to deal with what's ahead. And your family should be prepared as well.

If you take your parent into your home, you have to be prepared to have them stay with you for good, unless their health status changes to the degree that you cannot take care of them anymore. Then the need for hospitalization or nursing home placement may be the only way of providing appropriate care.

But if the move of your parent is not thought out fully, or is not working out despite your best intentions, or other members of your family are not happy with the arrangement, changes need to be made. If it is your parent who is unhappy with the situation of living in your home, then you should, with the approval of your parent seek out another residential option.

The situation becomes more problematic if it is not your parent that is unhappy with the situation, but it is your child or your spouse. If changes need to be made, and you need to ask your parent to move into another residential arrangement, the situation may become painful to your parent, as well as to you. Your parent may feel rejected, unwanted, unloved, and abandoned. He or she may also blame you for giving away their home, all or most of their belongings, and moving them in with your family when now you're about to move them again.

That it is why you should very carefully consider the option of bringing your parent to live with you and your family. But if the situation works, it is the most wonderful thing that a child can do for his or her parent. This option tends to be the least expensive option, of all other options. However, there is a price tag attached to this option as well.

Cost of Care

This chapter will present the cost issues for different settings, such as retirement communities and nursing homes. You have to remember that these costs are averages, and they do differ greatly from state to state. At our website www.goldeyearsgolden.com , as at the end of this book you will find contact addresses that will help you find the right facility and information regarding the cost in your state. Some of those options may or may not be covered by LTC insurance.

In simple terms LTC insurance can protect your assets and savings. It covers a wide variety of services. It can cover home care services, partially or fully. It can cover living facilities or nursing homes. Some insurance will cover safety modifications in the home of the insured, if it is required by the doctor. It may be as basic as bathtub or shower safety bars, hospital beds or ramps for wheelchairs. It all depends on the policy you have, and what it includes.

Reading the fine print of the insurance policy is a must. You want to make sure you know exactly what the policy covers, and more importantly, what it does not cover. You do not want any surprises down the road. Most policies will contain information as to what requirement they have before you can start collecting payment for long term care. Some may have a stipulation that for the first few months when you begin the use of long-term services, costs are not covered. Payment will kick in after that initial period.

As we know, the cost for long-term health insurance can be very high. Cost for nursing homes or residential care can wipe out even large savings. Most insurance does not totally cover the cost, and when savings are depleted, children step in to fill the gap if they can. But there aren't many children that can handle this burden over a long period. Today, more than 15 million children are taking care of their aging parents, paying for all or some of their housing expenses, as well as for their medical expenses. Some of the expenses are out of pocket and hard to keep track of. They may include the cost of home repairs, food, clothing, toiletries, small bills, and more. If you live far away from your parent, the costs can pile up even faster, due to the fact that it is harder to shop for better prices, or do comparative shopping.

According to a study done by AARP, most people have no idea how much it costs to provide LTC. Most Americans believe that Medicare provides for LTC, but it does not. It only provides for 100 days of rehabilitation.

Now that old people are living longer than they did generations ago, care must be provided on a longer basis, which makes the cost higher. Children are forced to supplement the cost for a parent's care, when at the same time they need to pay for their own children's education, and save for their own retirement.

As this book went to press, the children who pay a great deal for their parents' expenses are not able to deduct that expenditure on their taxes. As the costs escalate, and the baby boomers become a force to be reckoned with, I am sure the pressure will increase on elected officials to come up with some tax benefit, to ease the financial pain of children co-paying the cost of their parents' care.

As the cost skyrockets for LTC, lower cost options such as day care centers are becoming more popular, especially for patients with dementia, such as Alzheimer's, or patients who are limited in their mobility and require a great deal of assistance in daily activities. As diagnoses become more accurate, and the number of people needing those services is growing. Medicare does not provide coverage for most such needs. So if the person needing such a help, has LTC insurance, he or she has less to worry about.

So, if average cost of nursing homes hovers between $80,000 and $100,000 per year, and residential care cost can be around $50,000 a year, home care can run between $30,000 and $70,000, depending on the amount of coverage given. The need for LTC insurance becomes a no-brainer.

The cost of both the care and the insurance can vary from state to state. At the end of this book you will find addresses, as well as Web site links, that can help you find the information to help make the right decisions suited to your specific situation. But you will still need to do the research and comparison yourself.

Home care can be quite costly, but you can control the amount by using care as you need it. If you parent or loved one needs assistance for doctor appointments, or shopping, or some household tasks, you can pay just for that. You can add hours of care as the need presents itself.

The cost for one hour for a personal care aide (PCA) or home health aide (HHA) can range from $10 to $20. It varies from state to state, and from agency to agency; 24-hour coverage is billed as a flat fee by most agencies. This may cost you from $100 to $250 per 24 hours of care.

If your parent requires assistance due to illness or accident, Medicare will pay for it right out of the hospital if their doctor requests it. Medicare will provide coverage for only for a few weeks, and most of the time it will be limited to four hours per day. Most agencies will accept payment from Medicare for the four hours and then you will have to pay privately for whatever additional hours are needed.

Most agencies have a special fee schedule for 24-hour coverage or minimum number of days of coverage, thus lowering the hourly cost. In my agency, like with many other agencies, the cost of 24-hour coverage was equal to 13 hours. Check if the costs for home care in your state, when proscribed by your parent's doctor, is a recognized tax deduction for your parent.

LTC insurance could ease the pain of the cost. In the chapter on LTC insurance, we show the differences between several insurances. Keep in mind that the earlier one purchases such a policy, the lower the cost.

An average LTC insurance policy will cover a basic cost of around $200 a day in a nursing home; such a policy will cost in the around $2,500 per year when the policy holder is 55 years old, and around $4,000 when the policy holder is 65 years old. To lower the yearly cost of the LTC insurance, you may cut some of the benefits, for example if you take a policy that will cover three years in place of five years, the cost will be cut by nearly $500 per year for 65 year olds, and close to $1,000 for 55 year olds.

Retirement communities, also called senior citizens communities, may be the widest price range. You can find units ranging from the $20,000 into the millions of dollars. Here you really have to do your homework. You need to find the community that is in the area that is most suitable for your parent and within their financial ballpark.

Aside from the price tag attached to entering a retirement community, you should consider the location. If it is preferable that your parent lives near you, it will not help to find better priced places in other states, or even in distant communities in your state. It is hard to maintain a regular visitation schedule when your parent is far away.

One of the things you should consider to cut costs greatly is places that are partially financed by the state or federal government. You may consider renting a unit in such a community before buying to make sure that your parent likes living there. When looking at the price for such a unit, make sure you know of ALL costs.

Ask the following questions:

1. What is the full price for the unit?
2. What is the monthly cost if there is a mortgage?
3. What is the monthly maintenance fee?
4. What does the monthly maintenance include?
5. Can any other fees be added to the above?

6. What is the cost for a meal program?

7. How flexible is such program?

You would also like to know how difficult it is to sell the unit, if your parent is unhappy there or when she or he passes on. You may want to know what the restrictions are up front; it can be disheartening to discover such restriction in fine print at the time you need to sell the unit. As mentioned in the chapter on retirement communities, always demand that your parent be able to try the place for a month, to get a feel for the social environment, the services, and the quality of food, if it accommodates dietary needs, and it is to your parent's taste.

All kind of added fees may appear on your parent's monthly bill, including trivial requests like charges for exchanging one food for another. Added charges tend to be small and ambiguous and not easily noticed, so be very careful when checking monthly statements. Some places do not provide monthly statements, which makes it even harder to follow added charges.

My recommendation is to never to allow direct payment from a banking account. Not only are they difficult to check for added charges, but they are also hard to correct when an overcharge is found.

As old fashioned as it may sound, a paper trail is a very good thing to have, especially when you are controlling the account for your parent from a distance. And although most financial advisers will advise you to keep all documents and receipts for only seven years, a word from the wise is to keep them as long as your parent or loved one is alive.

I will take the chance of repeating myself and say that all documents, agreements, and contracts for your parent, or yourself, should be kept safe, and organized, to be available if any questioning is needed.

If you parent does not have any assets, and can show that he or she did not have and assets in the last three years, they may qualify for Medicaid, which will step in to pay for home care, at the patient's home, or in a nursing home. If you should pick the home care route, you have to take into account that there will be costs other than the home care services, including utilities, food and things such as detergent, soap, toilet paper, etc. With limited assets, your parent will qualify for food stamps, and possibly for other subsidies, which will help with monthly spending. But, you need to remember that regulations and availability of subsidies vary from state to state.

No matter what option your and you loved one pick, and however far away your parent will be, you have to set up a system of personal oversight. Whether it is you, or a friend, or a distant relative who visits your parent, the caregiver or givers, have to know that someone is checking in on them and the patient is protected.

While evaluating the options, one should develop a written record, putting down all possible foreseen and unforeseen expenses in each category. This will allow an accurate comparison, between the different options of residential situations, and how much you can get for yours, or your parent's, dollar. As with any legally binding document, make sure your attorney reviews it before you sign it.

Chapter 4 –
Insurance Options-
What We Have and What We Need.

Health Insurance in General

For many years we have been told that it is to our advantage to have private providers of health care, and not a system of universal health provided by the government. Since the days of President Nixon, the HMOs have taken hold of our health care, and their grip has been tightening ever since.

The lobbyists and the politicians beholden to the HMOs and the health insurance companies keep scaring us about how horrible it will be if the government is the one administrating a national health system. We will all suffer, unable to get the care we need, and wait for months to see the doctor, etc. Only the private insurance companies and the HMOs are able to care for us.

Oh, really?

Yet we do already have a functioning national health program - and it is administrated by the government. It functions quite well. Its name is Medicare. I don't think that it should be extremely complicated to extend this program to include health coverage for all Americans, young and old alike.

In such a system, all clinics, doctors, and other providers of services, will continue to provide services, but they will be paid from one source, the government. Because the source of payment is centralized, the cost of administration would go down quite a bit, and uniformity of the whole system would simplify the process.

As I have said before, we are already spending the money on the health system; it is just not doing what it should be for the money spent on it. It is not to say that the insurance companies should not make profit while providing coverage; it is the amount of profit that should be limited. The insurance companies are the middle man between the actual provider of health care services, such as the doctor or the hospital, and the patient needing that service, so it is unacceptable that the middle man dictate the level of cost or the type of service that the patient should receive.

The current system of health services delivery reminds me of a gas station attendant who fills your tank, and decides, at his own whim, how much gasoline he will fill in your car tank and how much he will charge you. And that decision is totally disconnected from the gasoline supplier's costs. I am not in favor of governmental control of all aspects of our life, but where health care is an issue, it is the government's responsibility to control the overcharges and haphazardly provided services. As stressed in the chapter on health insurance, the average American citizen, if lucky enough to have health insurance coverage, is overpaying for it, and in most cases is not covered for the value of the cost. In many cases, we find out the limitations of our coverage at some point when an emergency occurs.

There is no question that the health system in America needs a total makeover. Many Americans do not have any long-term insurance coverage, or the coverage that they have is not sufficient to cover all their health needs.

And even when they are covered with insurance that is considered fairly good, it does not necessarily provide them with safe and quality health services. The service your personal physician provides is consistently tied to the type of health insurance you have. This situation is frustrating to doctors and patients alike.

The health care system we now have is deficient in the best of cases. Being that it is not uniform in its standards, and each health provider sets up its own system and regulation, and rules, it may be as different as day and night from one provider to another.

It is essential that we develop a health care system that is patient-oriented and based on information sharing among the different health providing organizations, uniformity of prices for services - based on actual cost to the provider - and on fairness to the patient. Nationally set practices for prevention, test requirements, and generally accepted markers that when set off will require accepted treatment, should not have to be approved by bureaucrats' decisions. That's especially true when those decisions are based on the financial cost to the provider.

In a quality and client-centered health care system, medical care that is safe, efficient, provided timely and fairly to the patient will be the only way to care for all Americans. It is the right of every American to be provided with a fair and working health system.

Currently, health providers base their care on the cost to them today. Therefore they do not focus on keeping us healthy over the long run. Rather than prevent illness, the health insurance companies tend to postpone the prevention treatment to push it past the age of 65, when the patient will qualify for Medicare, and the burden of treatment will fall on the government, i.e., the taxpayer.

Unfortunately, by postponing active treatment, it causes the patient to develop serious conditions related to his or her illness, and complications that may even take the patient's life in the worst case scenarios. Even at best, it could affect his or her quality of life.

If, however, the providers of health care insure us for as long as we live, it is in their interest to keep us healthy for as long as we live. The key to all of this is preventative medicine, and educating us in the need to practice healthy lifestyle. Coordinating provision of health care services between all points of services, with the understanding that the patient is in the center of the formula, will enhance the level of care and render us healthier, and living longer as productive members of our society. There is also a need to provide better systems of information sharing among doctors, service providers, and the insurance companies.

Long-term Insurance-Do you need it and When.

Throughout our lives we seek out insurance coverage to protect ourselves and our belongings, such as our homes, our cars, and other property. We make sure that we have health insurance and life insurance to protect our loved ones. Over the years we adjust our insurance polices to reflect changes such as age, health status, riches, etc. We add coverage as we see the need. But many of us forget to foresee the need to purchase long-term care (LTC) insurance. This is currently provided to the lucky ones through Medicaid and Medicare.

It is clear that long term health insurance is a must for every retiree. The rapid growth of health care cost threatens the financial security of most people in that age group. About 20% of seniors' annual income is spent on health-related needs, that beyond the Medicare, co-pay - which is the major part of the bill. In 2002, Americans spent $139 billion on LTC, for people of all ages, which amounted to nearly 9% of all health-related spending.

LTC insurance pays for care provided at the client's home, as well as in any institutionalized setting, but you have to make sure that your particular policy will provide for the setting you choose. LTC insurance covers long-term needs, but it can also cover a week or two of home care after surgery. Most insurance policies have a cap on the number of days that the policy will cover.

As previously stated, the cost for residential care, assisted living, and nursing homes can range from $40,000 to $100,000 per year and even more; insurance is a must or you will deplete your savings and investments in no time. So purchasing an LTC insurance policy will protect one's assets.

LTC insurance can sometimes be purchased through health insurance companies via employment group insurance. Some employers will allow this, especially if the employee is young and the purchase will not increase the total health policy for the employer. In most cases, it is expected of the worker to pay additionally for the LTC insurance.

In any case, if you or your loved one is about to buy LTC insurance, ask the following questions:

a. Is the policy comprehensive, i.e., covers all levels of care, such as in the home, assisted living, or in a nursing home?

b. What is the daily limit?

c. Is there a 5% annually compounded benefit period, or a limited time benefit policy?

d. Is there a spousal discount?

e. Can you find a home health aide or a caregiver on your own, or do you have to go through an agency? If so, does the agency have to be licensed or certified?

f. Is the home benefit based on a daily, weekly, or monthly payment maximum?

g. If the benefit is not used, can it be used in the future?

If a person meets poverty standards, the government, under the Medicaid program will step in and cover long-term care. Most nursing homes accept Medicaid payment for the patient. At times, a person will enter a nursing home as a private paying patient, and when his or her funds are depleted, Medicaid steps in to pay.

It is essential that we make sure that our parent does not let the insurance policy lapse. We need to check that there is a provision in the policy that will cover home care. If they do not have such insurance, you need to check if it is possible to add home care to their insurance, even partially. A good rule of thumb is: Review your parent's insurance yearly to make sure it is adequate.

I have seen people continue to pay insurance for a spouse who died a few years back, or for a car they don't have anymore. The role of the insurance policy is to protect the insured from catastrophic expenses that can wipe out their lifetime savings in a very short time. So make sure you are on top of all insurance policies to see that they are adequate.

There are ways to ensure that the spouse remaining at home maintains most of his or her assets. One is to buy LTC insurance. The actual sales of LTC insurance have been dropping in the last few years. Although my feeling is that the baby boomers joining the seniors' ranks will change that trend. With increased advertising and knowledge, more of them will purchase LTC insurance. The earlier you buy long-term health insurance, the cheaper it is. By waiting with the purchase of the insurance, the cost is not the only factor that may work against you. You may get sick or disabled in later years, and if that occurs you are likely be rejected for coverage by many insurance companies.

Another option is to buy the newer combination of insurance, where you put a large amount of money into a cash value policy, with the right to withdraw 2 percent of the death benefits each year to cover nursing home and home care expenses. After your passing, your heirs will receive the remaining insurance proceeds tax free.

The last option is to tap into your home equity. This is basically a loan against your house. The older you are, the higher the loan that you may receive. You can think of it as a credit line. This is the reverse mortgage option: if you forfeit the house to the lender, your heirs will not inherit it.

Keep in mind than when shopping for insurance coverage, remember that the agent is a sales person, and his or her interest is to sell rather than to protect you or your parent. Make sure that your parent is not alone when the sales pitch is made. It's often hard for younger and sharper people to withstand the craftiness of some salespeople, let alone for the elderly.

Before signing any contract, make sure to check on the insurance company with the Better Business Bureau, and your state senior protection agency.

When purchasing insurance for a younger person, do the math as to how much it will cost you, for the years that you are not likely to use the insurance, and if it is financially more advisable to purchase a partial policy and add to it later on. If you're 45 years old, it is not likely that you will require home care any time soon, so you may want to purchase a policy that will pay out $100 per day, for perhaps 100 days. Such a policy will cost much less than, say, $250 per day for 2 to 3 years of coverage. But when you're 55 years old, you may want to add to the coverage, and thus having avoided the 10 years of higher cost.

Always evaluate the insurance, with what the different federal and state programs offer. For example: If Medicare provides every senior citizen with 100 days of rehabilitation, you would not need your insurance to provide you with that. So when purchasing new insurance, or reevaluating an existing policy for renewal, make sure you do not pay extra for this additional service. No insurance salesman will point this out to you, as it would cut their commission.

What one should remember is that rules and regulation change from year to year. You can check with your state offices on insurance issues. You can also check with Medicare and Medicaid offices and with state offices for the elderly. The offices of your senator and congressman can provide you with information on changes in the Medicare laws.

Some states also offer insurance policies, at times lower priced than those on the general market. See the phone numbers at the end of this book, listed by area of residence.

But, as with everything else in life, we should be very cautious when purchasing LTC insurance. I recall an article by Charles Duhigg in *The New York Times* on March 26, 2007 which addresses the problems the elderly have when they submit claims for long-term care. After paying for years to maintain LTC policies, when the time comes to activate those policies, the insurance companies decline over and over again, or take their sweet time to pay.

The article mentions the plight of one elderly lady Rose Derks, who purchased a long-term policy, so she would not be a burden to her children if she needed long-term care. She purchased the policy in 1990 with her hard- scraped money.

In May of 2002, after numerous hospitalizations, bouts of hypertension, and diabetes, Mrs. Derks agreed to move to an assisted-living facility. But when she filed a claim to her insurance company, they refused to pay. The insurance company claimed that Mrs. Derks waited too long to file the claim, and that the assisted living facility was not licensed, despite the fact that it was licensed by the state. Then, the insurance company claimed that Mrs. Derks was not sufficiently ill to justify that level of care, despite of letters provided to them by her personal doctor.

Mrs. Derks received many letters from the insurance company, at times contradicting themselves from one letter to the next. As of the date the article was written, she was yet to receive a payment.

As more and more Americans are purchasing LTC insurance, the insurance companies are developing procedures that make filing claims more and more difficult, and in some cases impossible to collect payment.

The article also reports that a "review of more than 400 of the thousands of grievances and lawsuits filed in recent years shows elderly policy holders confronting unnecessary delays and overwhelming bureaucracies. In California alone, nearly one in every four long-term claims was denied in 2005, according to the state."

The insurance companies, at times, make it almost impossible hard to collect on claims. They prolong the process by sending the insured the wrong forms, and then denying the claim because the claim was filed on the wrong form. Many times the claimant either gives up or eventually dies.

The best way to avoid the pain and suffering in fighting with the insurance company is to thoroughly check and research a policy before buying one from a company with very poor record. Always check if the insurance company you're considering is involved in lawsuits with their customers for refusal of payment. This can be verified through your state Office of the Aged (see information at the end of this book).

To conclude, although we need LTC insurance, until the time the government provides the Americans with nationalized health insurance, which hopefully would include LTC coverage, we should be very careful in whom we put our trust and money. So check, check, and check again, and compare as many insurance companies that you can, from all possible sources, such as friends, relatives, your doctor, or local social services offices.

Long Term Care- The pros and the cons

Our society's demand for long-term care (LTC) is constantly increasing. Almost every adult in this country will enter long-term care, or deal with a parent, friend or relative that will need of long-term care services.

Demographic studies show that 40% of all adults in the United States who live to the age of 65 will enter an LTC facility, or receive long term care at their home, before they die. But very few people actually know this fact, and very few are ready to deal with it emotionally or financially. And most are not ready to deal with the flawed system that we currently have in this country.

We should not be caught off guard, therefore it is important to prepare ourselves. The public needs to be educated to deal with a complex system, in which purchasing long term care insurance is only one component in a multi-faceted preplanning program.

LTC insurance today is not very well known, and most people, while planning for their retirement, do not factor in this type of insurance in their plan. Yet not having this single insurance, may wipe out all your savings quite fast. From experience in my agency, I've encountered over and over the misconception that many of the elderly thought that Medicare would cover their home care and nursing home cost.

Although LTC insurance covers home care as well as nursing home care, it is still used in most cases as a payment for a nursing home. Still, LTC insurance should provide for a safe and livable environment while providing the best personal care in other residential options, such as residential care facilities and assisted living.

When a person grows older, becomes frail, weak, increasingly disabled, or starts losing their mental abilities, it is not a happy situation. No matter how much personal care that individual will receive, we can assume that care will not reverse the process. Still, with proper care, much can be done to maintain quality of life and LTC can make the difference in one's life.

If we provide care that is geared to the specific needs and problems of a patient, we may slow down the progress of the illness which could render the person totally dependent on others. Those of us who will have LTC insurance for such services will have the protection of the ability to pay for such care, without worrying that it will wipe us out financially.

When considering LTC, first principle should be that the care provided should be designated to improve the quality of life of the patient. The care requires a combination of care that is based on compassion and competence.

Although most people will totally agree that such care is the right of the patient, it is more of a rarity than we realize. For one thing, such care has not been well rewarded financially, thus pushing the well qualified workers out of the profession.

Nursing homes have been in the media for years now, continuously having their shortcomings, cases of abuse, reduced quality of care, and poor physical surroundings documented. How many times have you heard someone say "I will never put my loved one in a nursing home"? Yet, when the time comes and you have no choice, you have to do just that.

Many of the nursing home owners have grown very wealthy, while their employees who have provided the care to our loved ones, have not been paid a decent remuneration. Not only are the health aides that provide day-to-day care to the sick and disabled in the long-term institutions paid poorly, their profession does not provide them with much social respect. If we are to expect to bring into the field more qualified and dedicated workers, we will have to reward them with better pay and benefits, as well as with more respect and recognition.

So if you purchase LTC insurance make sure it will adequately cover the cost for the care, and then also check the particular institution that you are interested in to see if their workers are paid well and how great their turnover is. I always thought that I could identify unhappiness in the faces of the workers. Poor pay and disrespect can surely by seen on their facial expression. But more checking should be done, to verify the situation in the facility that you are considering in for your loved one.

The next thing you should look at before deciding on which health care road you pick is the following:

a. Determine the cost of the care giving, either at home or in a nursing home or any other health care facility.

a. Establish if the elderly has financial resources to provide sufficient funds to cover the LTC.

b. The cost of the care should be discussed with the elder, if she or he is mentally able to deal with the issue. This should be done discreetly and delicately, as many elderly have difficulties dealing with financial issues.

c. If it is at all possible, include other siblings into the structure of helping your parent or relative, thereby making the burden lighter on the parent or yourself.

LTC in this country was not a planned industry; it simply evolved. It come into being to fill a gap where the family could not provide for the daily care of the sick and disabled seniors, whose conditions were either not acute enough or chronic enough for hospital care. The irony is that today, it is so profitable to care for the old and chronically ill, that many hospitals go into the nursing home business and develop nursing homes on site or near by. There is money to be made from both ends billing the patient or the government or whoever pays for the care.

What came in to being as a very small business, something just to fill a narrow need in our changing society, turned to be a much bigger business when more financing became available.

The biggest reason for the change was the creation of Medicaid in 1965. The sudden influx of money into LTC, specifically nursing homes, brought desirability to the business of LTC.

Initially, nursing homes were babysitting facilities that essentially provided basic care for its residents. They fed, housed, and provided some personal care, such as bathing and assisting in dressing, as per the need. It was the equivalent of boarding houses.

The introduction of Medicaid changed the practices of housing the elderly, and maintaining them in those situations until their death. With Medicaid paying the bill for LTC, the designers of this program had never expected it would be a major vehicle to cover nursing homes.

The developers of the Medicaid program envisioned it to provide the elderly and the needy with coverage periodically and temporarily. They thought it would help mothers and children in need, maybe more than the elderly, who were financially unable to provide for themselves.

Being that the poorest segment of our society at the time of the formation of Medicaid, in the mid-'60s, were the elderly, and sick, the program evolved somewhat differently, and to a greater size than originally intended.

The federal government was caught unaware of the demographics and by the cost of the program. Re-evaluation needed to be done quickly. It needed to develop a frame work for the program, new ways to administer the program, and establish a new set of rules by which we admit the ones most needing help. The need to evaluate and set guidelines to foresee and minimize possible abuse of the program became necessary.

The available regulations that were in place at the time were for small hospitals. The government, for lack of any others, used those regulations for developing nursing home guidelines.

A major issue was safety: there was a need to establish safety guidelines in nursing home care and adapt them unilaterally throughout the field. After this was done, most nursing homes ended up resembling small hospitals.

In spite of nursing homes being treated like small hospitals at the time, there were significant differences between them. Small hospitals provided more acute care, on a mostly short-term basis. As far as the nursing home care, it was supposed to provide the closest possible environment to being home. It was presumed that it would be a social environment and socially stimulating. The reality was somewhat different through the early years; the long-term institutions were just that, institutions. A patient's individuality had little room in the nursing homes at that time.

When one enters a hospital, one agrees to give up one's, identity and individuality, even if it's only temporary. One's dignity and control over their life is temporarily suspended, in lieu of a reasonable hope and expectation that one will get better.

One endures the indignity of wearing those terrible hospital gowns, making an individual become just like all the rest of the patients, with no sense of individuality and almost no say as to what it is that is done to them. One is woken up at all hours of the night, not always for obvious reasons. In most cases, one shares a room with a stranger, who might be sicker or noisier. And one is willing to suffer all this indignity, and will forgive it all, in exchange for improved health.

Now, when you think of it, the deal in a nursing home is much worse. Most people entering a nursing home will, in all likelihood stay there until they die. It is basically their last home. The physical environment is basically the treatment. Not surprisingly, not too many people rush to enter into nursing homes. If the elderly has any other choice, he or she will not likely choose a nursing home. Nursing homes seem to be the last refuge.

For a long time, the public policy was looking for alternatives to the nursing home option. First, looking within the community, by supporting home care, where the patient receives assistance in his or her home. More recently, through supporting some assisted living facilities that provide different degrees of assistance.

In this climate, it is understandable why assisted-living facilities have sprung up by the thousands, like mushrooms after a rain. Private investors, as well as all sorts of organizations, such as religious, professional and other organizations, saw this area as having a potential for profit-making as well as the chance to provide care to specific population groups that are of interest to their organizations.

At the initial stages of establishing assisted-living facilities, the provision of services was basically based on provision of hotel services, rather than a health care model. The original concept of assisted living was designed based on the need to address the deficiencies and the shortcomings of the nursing home system, the worst of which was the lack of respect to the privacy and individuality of the residents.

So, with each wave of new assisted-living institutions, there would be the offer of new variations. It did not take long before the name "assisted- living facility" lost any meaning. Almost any type of housing that is shared in any way and provided some form of services, no matter how limited, was called assisted-living facility.

Because both the nursing homes and assisted living serve similar populations, there was a need to set up new policies and regulations to protect the residents. The need to maintain standards became clear, after many scandals erupted in the 70s, and deficient care was shown in many nursing homes.

Those, scandals brought to the public's attention the possibility of abuse of the very people who need our protection the most, a population very susceptible to abuse. It became politically necessary to establish unifying regulations, and some kind of licensing to regulate the field of assisted living, as well as to establish tougher demands on the owners and administrators of nursing homes.

When interviewing people who are working actively in the nursing home field, some maintained that all the added regulations and restrictions helped to shape the nursing homes into institutions that became very impersonal. Due to overregulation, residents' needs were pushed to the bottom line and what was actually good for them was lost

On the other hand, others in the field maintained that residents are only protected from abuse, inappropriate care, and deficient treatment in the nursing home by those regulations. It has to be understood that without such regulations and guidelines, the elderly residents of such institutions would be at the mercy of the providers. If the owner/provider is a good and caring person, the care may be good, or satisfactory. But what if the provider is just in it for the financial gain and the wellbeing of the patient is secondary to him?

One may ask why both assisted living and nursing homes should be held to the same standards. They each provide different services for different populations. The two also provide different levels of services. There are of course some similarities; they each fill a niche that provides needs that the resident requires.

Some of the services overlap at times, but as a rule of thumb, the nursing homes provide care to people with more acute health issues. In the assisted living institutions, the residents are at a higher level of functionality. They are able to perform all their basic needs on their own, without assistance. They can bathe, dress, and feed themselves.

On the other hand, they do need help with shopping, cooking, cleaning, and laundry. That is why assisted living is more appropriate for them. It also fills their social needs and they do not need to live alone.

Assisted living facilities are currently turning their marketing to look to the potential market of the future, people in their fifties. The targeted markets of potential residents are quite autonomous, but ultimately do not want the burden of running their own household.

The assisted living facilities range from very basic, that of providing living quarters with hotel-like services, to very opulent residential situations with recreational opportunities and gourmet food with five-star restaurant services.

Originally the assisted-living facilities were built around high-functioning residents, and when the resident's condition changed and their health status reduced his or her level of independence requiring an increased level of care, the resident was transferred to a nursing home.

The assisted living business became so profitable, that the owners and organizations running them are developing sections in them to allow the provision of a higher level of health care services.

Some will allow the family to bring a personal caregiver, rather than gradually extend the level of care and services; other assisted-living facilities have contracts with home care agencies that will provide a home care aide to cover the needs of the resident. This service is paid by the resident separate from the cost of the assisted living.

Only when the resident's condition requires continuous medical care, is the resident transferred to a nursing home. In general there is an understanding that most assisted-living facilities try to maintain an energetic and upbeat atmosphere in their facility. I have visited assisted- living facilities that did not allow wheelchairs, and residents with disabilities, such as blindness, were discouraged to apply; of course this is done subtly.

The option of assisted living is an expensive one. The assisted living idea is basically recreating the home care situation, in a shared-living environment.

Financing sources are different for the two options. The nursing home stay is, to a large extent financed by Medicaid, if the elderly qualifies due to lack of funds. Some elderly initially start off paying privately until their funds are depleted, and than Medicaid steps in. To a smaller degree, private insurance is also a source of payment, if the senior has such a policy covering them for nursing home stay. And the rest is private pay.

The assisted living option is mostly financed privately. Some insurance policies will provide partial financing for assisted living, but policies tend to be expensive, and at times very vague as to under which conditions it will pay its portion for assisted living. You should make sure when purchasing such a policy, to be fully informed as to which facilities of assisted living the policy will provide payment, if it has any restrictions and conditions under which it will not pay for such service.

You should make sure that you clearly understand the insurance policy restrictions on assisted living facilities, and if they need to be licensed by state or federal agencies, if they need to show any specific qualifications, etc. You do not want to discover all these restrictions after your parent is admitted to an assisted living facility and moved in. If the payment is rejected by the insurance company, you are left holding the bill.

A growing number of states are beginning to finance some portion of the assisted living cost. But it is still a small part of the bill. The cost of assisted living may force the family to decide between the more socially and satisfactory way of life, and the cheaper less desirable way of living in a nursing home, which in most cases is covered by government programs such as Medicaid.

For a very long time the care in long-term facilities was substandard. Maybe that was due to the fact that our expectations were very low.

Choices were limited and one was thankful to be able to find a place for his mother or father, and quite afraid to "rock the boat," so to speak, for fear of losing a place for their loved ones.

But with time, nursing homes did change the quality of care they provide. I will not argue that there still much to be done to improve them, but all the rules and regulation that were developed and the oversight by different governmental agencies eliminated abuse and placed the responsibility on the providers, making them accountable if such mistreatment should occur.

As the number of chronically ill and frail seniors continues to increase, there is a need to establish appropriate facilities that will provide human and quality health and personal care. The cost should also be at a level that is manageable by the individual applying for the service.

When taking into account the whole picture of LTC, the government should plan and project for the future cost of providing the aforementioned quality and availability. The cost for such care is already very high and is going to rise much higher, unless we revamp the total structure of LTC.

If given the choice, most people would choose to stay in their own home, or have the combination of home stay with the support of home care, to varying degrees, with the support of the family - either directly providing the care or arranging and paying for the care provided by agencies, and overseeing the quality of care.

Home care cost should be evaluated versus the cost of institutionalized care, when the cost is borne by the public. But the cost should not be the sole factor on which the decision is made regarding the source of care.

And although we would all likely agree with the notion that the provision of homecare is by far the best choice, there comes a time that institutionalized care may be the better option. What we should do is to make sure that the care provided in such communal situation is up to par and care is administered in a more efficient way.

It will be quite a challenge to design, and develop a health system that provided the needed care to the recipient in their own home, but more so in an institutionalized setting or in any other shared residential setting. It is important that the rights of the recipient are not overshadowed in the process of receiving the said care.

LTC should be brought to the forefront of the political agenda. We should demand our elected officials to push LTC to the top of their agenda. The sheer numbers of the seniors carry great power, and it is important to use that power for the benefit of the seniors themselves.

All these changes should be implemented now. We cannot postpone them into the far future. The elderly need them today. Increased quality of care brings with it increased quality of life.

By improving the provision of LTC, we improve not only the quality of life of the person receiving the care, but also that of their family and society in general is better off when its elders are well cared for.

And it should be understood by all that it is not necessary to make a trade off between quality of life and quality of care. We need to encourage broader coverage, separate the cost and payment for services from the room and board. A person should be able to receive the same high quality of care, regardless of in which residential situation he finds himself. The same services should be provided and paid for if he lives in his home, a nursing home, a residential care facility, or an assisted-living environment.

If a system like the one described above is developed, it will be based on the above-mentioned options, meaning that all medical and health-related services will be accessible to a person if he or she will stay in their home, if that is what they desire. But if their condition dramatically changes, it will mandate that they would be moved into some sort of communal setting, such as a nursing home or residential facility. That residential change would mean no change in the quality of health and medical services they require.

We should not only encourage the institution of broad practices of high quality of care, we should demand it. Regulations, old and new, should be revisited and adapted to reflect the present-day situations. It should be understood that safeguards for quality of care must not be compromised.

Most people in need of LTC tend to have multiple health issues, at times requiring multi faceted medical care. We need to set up ways to provide uninterrupted venues of medical care to people receiving LTC. The system needs to be simplified, to allow the seniors and the elderly to easily navigate it. It should be easily understood, with clear directions of expectation.

Although it is a complex issue, LTC should and can be provided universally. Countries poorer than the United States have been providing these services for a long time. We know it is possible, but how we pay for it is the question. The money needed to universally provide LTC can come from public funds, through the government, and from the private sector.

It is morally right to provide for our elders as they deserve the care; they paid into the system, and it is their right for the system to pay into them.

Medical Coverage-Are you insured

Over the years many politicians have declared that every American is entitled to medical coverage that will provide him or her with all their health needs. But for some reason, as soon as they are elected to the Senate or Congress, all those promises and declarations are forgotten. Ironically the people who have the power to decide if and when we, the American people, will be covered by universal medical coverage, are themselves covered by excellent medical coverage.

Both senators and congressmen choose from a wide variety of medical insurance plans, through the Federal Employees Health Benefit Program. There are doctors and nurses actually working in the Capitol. There is a small pharmacy available to the members to pick up their medication. An outstanding military hospital located not far from the Capitol is also available to them, if more serious health issues require treatment.

The very people we elect to represent us, do very well for themselves, and often forget about the very people who elected them, leaving us to continue to struggle with no or insufficient medical insurance coverage.

In 2008, the Democratic presidential candidates all presented plans for a national medical insurance coverage, some more and some less extensive. Any coverage would be welcomed and better than what we have currently.

We continually hear that universal health coverage cannot be realistically put into place because of the massive cost. The truth is that we are already spending the money; it just needs to be allocated into the right places. And as I already stated, the government should put limits on profits that the insurance companies are making. As un-American as it may sound, regulations are needed because the profit-seeking is what makes the cost of medical insurance so high.

It is time that every elderly, middle-aged, and young American received full medical coverage, without worrying that an illness might wipe them out financially, or that they would wind up with a life threatening illness because they were unable to afford preventive treatment.

Many working Americans who annually earn more than $30,000 or $40,000 are living without medical insurance. They would gladly pay for medical insurance if they could afford it. This would be possible if the cost of insurance coverage came down; it would not only allow a great many of the 47 million Americans that are currently uninsured to purchase medical coverage, but it actually would be financially beneficial.

To decrease medical costs, better emphasis should be made on educating the population through many channels to practice better health habits. We can start as early as kindergarten, with teaching children proper hygiene and washing hands. Older children can be taught better eating habits, to avoid smoking, and to engage in physical activities on a regular basis. Most importantly, preventive medicine - including regular checkups and seeing doctors at the earliest stages of an illness - will prevent more costly treatment when untreated illness becomes more complicated.

So you may ask yourself why there is no bigger outcry from Americans demanding the obvious: health coverage to all. In my opinion it is simple because we have been brainwashed for so long to think that if the government took over the health system, the quality of the care would suffer or the costs would bankrupt us.

The Americans who are covered by insurance companies, however insufficient that coverage may be - with payments of ranging from $350 to $1000 per month and out-of-packet co-pays constantly rising, are afraid to rock the boat, fearing that providing all Americans with medical insurance will raise their own costs. This fear comes from misconceptions and misinformation. The fact is that the uninsured population seeks out health services to a great extent from hospital emergency departments. The hospitals are required by the government to provide 10 percent of their care to the poor and uninsured. The cost for such care is already factored in the cost of insurance you are paying.

The biggest percentage of the money in the health insurance pot goes to bureaucracy and profit. As for the cost of the actual care provided to the patient, those services have unfortunately become a product subject to market forces. Hospitals became corporations that concentrate more on their bottom line rather than on the patient. The patient is a source of income, and how the cost is ultimately bourn is secondary.

When admitted to the hospital, the patient is put through many tests, some of which may be unnecessary. There are several reasons for this, including the presence of "good insurance" policy and the constant fear of malpractice lawsuits. All possible tests are done so there is no base for negligence.

If the general population, including both the insured and uninsured, understood that it is to their benefit to join in demanding fair and equal coverage for everyone, a movement to establish such insurance might actually take hold.

And until that time, even though you may think that you are fully insured, you are still at the mercy of your medical insurance provider.

Case # 8

This story still breaks my heart every time I think about it. It happened to friends of mine, two hard working people, about twenty five years ago. Both held what we would consider good jobs with good pay and very generous benefits, including excellent medical coverage provided by the employer.

My friends were well on their way to fulfill the American dream, with a little house, two children, and annual vacations. As a young family, they considered themselves very lucky, but then tragedy struck. Their ten- year-old son was diagnosed with ADL, a debilitating and terminal illness that took his life four years later.

Initially, the little boy's care was fairly simple, consisting of regular visits to the doctor. A year later he required assistance with activities of daily living, as his motor skills began to fail. As the illness progressed, and the child lost the ability to ambulate, became incontinent, and needed home care, the insurance company began to reject the bills. The father, whose insurance coverage was being billed, was called in to his boss's office, and apologetically informed that they have no choice but to let him go. Otherwise, the company will loose the health policy for the whole company of some 80 workers, and the cost for the policy would go up so much that wouldn't be able to afford it.

So my friend, not only lost his health coverage, he also lost his job. All this happened as my friends were in a heart-wrenching race to find something that would slow down the illness from robbing their son's ability to walk, to talk, to see, and eventually to live. For part of the care, the wife's insurance stepped in and covered the expenses; unfortunately her medical insurance was not as good as her husband's, and had high co pays.

For the next two years, the care for the little boy advanced to feeding through G-Tube, which required special care and supplies. His home care was extended to 24 hours per day with aides coming and going, and nurses visiting to provide daily care, such as medication to deal with reoccurring infections that he was unable to fight. They fought with him and for him for the next two years, until his untimely passing. In the process this fight depleted their savings, and forced them to slowly sell off whatever they had of value until they sank under the debt.

I was so naïve at the time. I actually thought that the insurance companies were there to help you, that if you or your employer pays for years for medical coverage, they would be there for you when you need them, especially in the cases of serious illness. But some insurance companies are there to take your money, and when the need occurs, they will do anything to avoid paying.

My friends still have not recovered from the loss of their child, or from the financial loss, for that matter.

Medical Treatments Abroad

Just like the population at large, many seniors do not have any health insurance. But unlike younger members of the population, most seniors are entitled to Medicare coverage when they reach the qualifying age. Still, even with Medicare, they need to pay out of pocket for medical care. If the medical need is an emergency, a surgical procedure, or a serious chronic or terminal illness, the 20 percent of your co-pay alone may be so costly that it can wipe out your savings in no time.

The choices for medical coverage are currently private medical insurance coverage - whether partial or full - supplemented with Medicare, after qualifying. If a person has just Medicare coverage and no financial resources, he will qualify for Medicaid coverage, with or without Medicare.

Sadly many seniors, even those covered by medical insurance, are not able to receive the full medical treatment they need. At times the out-of-pocket co-pay forces the senior to forgo the treatment. The fragmentation of our medical coverage, with approval and payment for medical services coming from different sources, sometime leads to insurance companies go back and forth, trying to have the "other" sources pay for the medical services, leaving the patient vulnerable.

For some time now, Americans have been seeking medical and dental treatments from other countries, such as Thailand, India, Costa Rica, Brazil, South Africa, Romania, Hungary, and other eastern European countries. More than a half million Americans have received overseas medical care, by choice, last year. This is the result of the high cost of medical insurance, and the resulting deficiencies in coverage.

Medical care and specific surgical procedures, such as open heart surgery, joint replacement surgery, cosmetic surgery, back surgery, etc., are geared to the American public, frequently including swanky accommodation..

Overseas medical care is provided, for the most part, by staff that is fluent in English, and many of the doctors have been educated or trained in their specialties in the United States. Most of the time, these procedures cost less than 50 percent as the same procedure done in the United States.

The international medical provision of specific treatments is usually well organized, with representation in the United States. If you choose to be treated in one of those countries, you will be instructed as to special traveling arrangements, hotels for recuperation stay, pickup from the airport, and transportation upon return.

There are people who highly recommend going overseas for medical treatment. Still my recommendation would be to be careful in researching the hospitals and clinics, before setting out to put your life and health into their hands. You could check for accreditation with the International Joint Commission, or the World Health Organization (WHO), but even if the places check out with those agencies, you may want to research the institutions' background, accreditations and personnel qualifications on the internet. Your doctor also should be included in the decision-making.

Some private insurance companies will pay for some of such out-of-country medical treatment; in most cases it is cheaper for them than to pay for the same procedure done in the U.S.. You should check with your insurance company to see if they will cover it. Even with all the cost of traveling and the expense of hotels, you may still come out ahead than the co-pay you would have to pay here.

The drawbacks for such a choice are few, but they are of high importance and one should consider them, before choosing medical care abroad. Upon return, who is going to provide you with follow up care? That is by far the most important reason why your doctor at home should be part of the decision to seek medical care abroad. If at all possible, the doctor performing the medical procedure should communicate with your doctor at home.

The other drawback is in case of problems arising from the procedure, due to negligence or error on the part of the staff, you would have limited, if any, legal recourse. Being alone in a strange country, you are totally dependent on people you don't really know. Suppose you arrive at your destination, after paying for all or part of the procedure, and you discover that the medical staff is unprofessional and unqualified, or the facility is not what was presented to you before you arrived. Well, you would have a hard time recouping your payment, and would have to turn around and return home. You need to also know, that most of the foreign medical facilities do not carry malpractice insurance.

If you will decide to go that route, or if you do not have another choice, you should consider the following to guide you and help you to prepare for such a trip.

First, seek advice from your private physician; he or she may be knowledgeable on the subject, and may advise you directly or refer you to sources that may help you to become better informed and prepared to make your decision. Try to talk to specialists in the United States as to their thoughts about doing the procedure in the particular country you are considering.

You should educate yourself on the subject, especially about your type of medical need. The Internet is a great source for that. How many procedures like the one you need does the facility do a year? What is their rate of success? If an implant is used during the procedure, check what kind it is, the implant's safety record, and if it's standard is up to par with the same implant used in the United States.

Find out if you can make arrangements through a health travel agency. Those agencies can find medical destinations for you that will reflect your needs. But you should know that sometimes the agency also represents the medical facility, thus their recommendations may be biased.

Make sure that you know all the costs involved, and you have the price in writing, with no hidden costs. Financial arrangements should be clear, in writing, and the method of payment should be clearly understood.

Take all medical records relevant to your condition such as letters from your doctors, reports of all tests that have been done, x-rays, MRI, CT scans, etc., with you. On the way home, bring back with you all medical records that contain all the information regarding the procedure for your personal doctor to review.

If at all possible bring a family member or a friend with you, to advocate for you in case of need, especially if the procedure you are having renders you unable to make decisions for yourself.

You can speak with the doctor over the phone prior to going overseas, so you develop a rapport with the doctor who will provide the care that you seeking so far away from home.

Check with your insurance if they will cover the procedure fully or partially when it is done abroad. Make sure that you have the commitment from the insurance company in writing. This will eliminate misunderstanding later on, when the time comes to be reimbursed.

Let's hope that in the future there will be no need to seek health care outside the borders of our country.

No one in his right mind will dispute the fact that our country is blessed with one of the best medical health systems in the world, and it will be wonderful to have it accessible to every American, young, old, and in between. Let's hope.

Chapter 5 –
Drugs and Documentations-
The "D's" That Keep You Well.

Prescription Drugs-Learn how to save

Through the Medicare Part D plan you are entitled to receive your prescription medication at a reduced fee. In the chapter dealing with Medicare you will find information dealing specifically with Medicare Part D, but in this chapter I'd like to touch on prescriptions drugs in general.

When you are prescribed medication by your doctor, you should check the prices of the medication you need at your local pharmacies. You'd be surprised at the price range you will find.

The option of generic medication is becoming more and more appealing. Using generic drugs can cost you at times 75 to 80 percent less per prescription. As commonly known, many of the brand medications are losing their patent protection, allowing the generic market to grow and produce duplicates of those medications. Billions dollars worth of brand name medication are losing their patent protection in the coming years, allowing us to purchase generic medication at just a fraction of the cost.

If you are using a brand medication, and there is no generic drug equal to it, ask your doctor if there is a generic drug that is similar which may be used for your specific needs. The use of generic drugs will be financially beneficial.

If you are insured by an HMO or other health insurance company like I am, you in all likelihood have a co-pay with your prescriptions.

Your co-pay may have three levels, for example - $10, $25, and $50 - with the lowest being the co-pay for generic drugs.

Insurance companies devise all sorts of prescription plans, such as mail-order services for your medications or the option to order a three-month supply at once, to get your medication at reduced price. Then there is the Wal-Mart program, with the 30-days supply of medication offered for $4. The medications are all generic and the list of the medications is not very long. Target, another retail chain store, also offers some 315 different medications for $4. And Walgreen's Drug stores offers 90-day supplies of some 300 generic drugs for the reasonable fee of $12.99.

Some other mega-store chains have jumped into the game too. Costco, had tried the $4 prescription model, but ended up switching to a price of $10 for 100 pills. A regional supermarket chain, Giant Eagle, currently offers some 400 generic drugs for $4 each, and Meijer, another chain of stores, offers the seven most common antibiotics for free. It would be nice to see other chains to join these ranks.

More than half of the medications being used today are for chronic illnesses. Because those medications are taken over long periods of time, one can order the supplies for 90 days and save some money. And some of the suppliers will ship the medication free of charge. The deals vary from one plan to another; some will mail you medication for three months' use and charge you just for two months. So check with your health insurance plan and see if it is something you can benefit from.

It is advisable to make sure that all suppliers are within the United States and comply with FDA regulations. When ordering from abroad you do not know if you are actually getting what you ordered and if the medication is safe.

The cost of the co-pay on your prescriptions, as well as any other out-of-packet cost of medication' may be applied to your medical expenses when doing your taxes. Check with your accountant if you use a great deal of medication, since the deduction may be significant.

Medication and the Elderly

One of the most important issues in the care of the elderly is to establish safety guidelines for the use of medication. Regardless of where one resides and her or his medical status, we should be cognizant of the seniors' ability to follow their medications routine and to their ability to follow their doctor's instructions.

If the elderly person lives in an assisted-living facility, a residential care facility, or a nursing home, his or her medications are dispensed by a nurse according to their doctor's orders. But when they administer it to themselves it can be a concern.

Many seniors who live on their own forget to take their medications on time, and do not follow their doctors' directions. At times they forget if they took their medication and then repeat their dose. Some of them confuse one medication for another, and take inappropriate doses.

When a senior receives home care by a qualified home care aide, the aides are trained to prompt the senior to take the right medication at the right time. The home attendant will also be able to see if there are any allergic reactions to medication and alert the patient's doctor, informing the doctor of what symptoms the patient experienced.

It is the senior that lives on his or her own, and administers their medication independently, that is the real issue here. They visit doctors, and are often rushed in and out without understanding all that the doctor requires them to do. And if they do not write it down, there is a chance that they will forget what is required of them.

For example if the doctor says a medication is to be taken before eating, or with food, or after meals, it is hard for an elderly person to remember, especially if they have a number of medicines, for different illnesses and conditions, and each medication has a different set of instructions as to the way it should be taken.

If the senior has a family member, a friend, or a person who is involved in their care, they should help to set up a system for safe administration of medication.

There are few ways of doing it, and at times, the best system is found by trial and error. You can choose the method that is most suitable for you or for your loved one. Weekly pill boxes have daily compartments, and medication is set up for the whole week. If all the medication is taken at the same time on a daily basis, you can purchase a seven-day box with only one compartment per day; if medication is to be taken a few times a day, there are medication boxes with up to four compartments per day. The compartments are marked by day, for example, Monday, and then each daily compartment is marked:

morning, lunch, evening, and night. Medication is usually allocated weekly, so it is necessary to make sure that enough medication is on hand to do that.

What I like about the medication box is that a great deal of guessing is eliminated. All you have to do is check the appropriate box to find out if you forgot to take the medication. It happens to me more often that I would like to admit: that I question myself: did I take my medication?

If the elderly is living on their own and does not have home health services or a relative or friend to come in and allocate the medication for the week, they can take the medication and the medication box to be filled for the week by the nurse at their doctor's office. Most doctors' staff will help with that task.

A visiting nurse can also be arranged through private insurance, as well as through Medicare and Medicaid.

The medication boxes have another benefit: they are easier to open, than the pharmacy-supplied medication containers, which can be difficult to open even by people that do not have arthritis and other joint problems.

It is very important to have an up-to-date list of medication printed clearly and posted in a very visible place like the refrigerator; the list should include not only the name of the medication, but the dosages and the times it should be taken. And nothing is easier than to check the compartment if you're not sure if in fact you did take the medication.

A copy of a current medication list should be kept with any person who is taking any prescribed medication, either in their handbag or their pocket. It is essential that one takes that list to any doctor appointment, and shows it to the doctor, so there can be an evaluation if there is a need to continue with the medication, if the dosage remains unchanged, or if new medication needs to be introduced. The doctor has so many patients and does not always clearly know what you are already taking. With our care fractioned by so many different specialists, and each prescribing different medications, it is very important that they all know what is prescribed to you by other doctors.

Another method that I have seen seniors use is a daily list, where each medication is listed, along with the time of taking. After taking the medication the senior marks the space next to the medication that he or she has taken it. This system requires some record keeping, and either the senior or someone else needs to prepare the forms, but it does provide a paper trail for medication taking.

Family members, care givers, or doctors need to be cognizant to the fact that some times the elderly will not take their medications as prescribed Trying to save money; they may periodically skip a dose, thinking it won't cause problems, to make the medication last longer.

The key is that medication should be taken to help, not to hurt you. Proper usage of medication is required, as well as good coordination between the different doctors that prescribe the medications and take care of you and your loved one.

Case # 9

Mr. B. was an independent elderly gentleman that called our agency, asking us to help him out five hours a day, seven days a week - just with care of the house chores, assisting him with shopping, food preparations, and escorting him to doctor visits.

He was independently handling his relationship with the doctor, as well as his medication administration. When we came in to provide the services, Mr. B. was evaluated by our nurse. Her perception was that his memory had been failing him, and that he could have some underlying medical problems that he either was not forthcoming about or was unaware of.

We asked to speak to his doctor, as per our requirements, to which he readily agreed.

Mr. B.'s doctor was quite happy that we came into the picture, because he too was apparently aware that Mr. B. had been slipping mentally, as well as physically. One of the things that the doctor was worried about was whether or not Mr. B. was taking his medication appropriately.

The doctor informed us that in the last year Mr. B. had come to him with symptoms that were consistent with taking medication inappropriately.

Considering that we only provided Mr. B. with five hours of services, it was important to establish a routine where most medication was taken during the hours the aide was there. Although Mr. B. did not initially want to let someone else make decisions for him, he slowly let go, as the doctor and the nurse from the agency worked out a routine that was safe. Medication was given with breakfast, when his aide started her day of work, and then again with lunch, before the aide left.

For the next two years we provided home care to him and he seemed to have improved - his life became more social, he was less forgetful, his memory improved, he ate better and slept better. Even more noticeable his bouts of agitations decreased, and his disposition improved.

Clearly, some of the symptoms Mr. B. was experiencing were directly related to taking medication inappropriately, and not following the directions given by his doctor. When Mr. B. had been taking medication incorrectly, he did not always remember whether he had taken the medication or not and often took a double dose. He did not understand why he was feeling sluggish, sleeping a great deal, his memory was failing him, and he was suffering from other symptoms, all of which cleared up after we straightened out the medication issue.

Documentation & Medical Records

As we age and more conditions affect us, the more specialists we see and the more there medical documents represent our medical history, the treatments we go through, and the medications we've taken.

The problem is that in most cases, all this documentation is in the hands of more than one doctor. If you had any hospitalizations or emergency room visits, your records are in the hospital. If you have a condition that requires the care of a specialist, he or she will have your records. If you require multiple specialists, each one will have your records related to the treatment they provide.

In the best of cases, they are in communication with each other, and each is aware of what the other is doing, especially concerning the medication they individually prescribe for you, so they are not contraindicated, doing you more harm than good.

With all the medical care that the average patient receives, through specialists and sub specialists, there is much room for errors, misdiagnosis, and possible unnecessary treatments.

This basically leaves the responsibility up to you to gather all your medical records, be educated about your illnesses, and read up on the medications you are taking, including the side effects. It is, after all, your life that it is in those records.

You should ask your doctors for all reports, tests, and copies of letters that doctors send to one another. And it is your right to receive a copy of all medical documents that pertain to you. It may even keep you healthier. After all, you are the only one of you that you have. To the doctor, as much as he or she may like you personally, you are one of many and it is hard for the doctor to keep track of every detail. That is where the records come in. Your doctor has a set, and you should too.

Today most records can be kept in electronic form, but systems are different, so most doctors keep a paper file of their patient's records. You basically can keep your own records, in any manner that is convenient, as long as you have copies.

The best way to keep your records is in a chronological order, with the most current on top; but there are other methods which you may want to check out at www.myphr.com. Among your medical records should also be a current printout from your pharmacy with a current list of all medications that you are taking.

When going to a new doctor or a specialist who does not know you or your medical history, bring your medical file to inform the doctor of your medical issues, what treatments you had or are having, and what medications you are taking. When you are prescribed a new medication, show the doctor a list of the medications you are currently taking, and ask if there is any issue with taking the new medication with the others you already are taking.

Keep your medical file in a place that is known to others, so that it can be found easily in times of emergency.

You should also keep a list of all the doctors that you are using for your health care. Write a short description of each doctor's specialty, making it clear to someone else if they read the file. Also list each doctor's name and telephone number, so it is available in an emergency.

It is also advisable to have a personal file, which will include your personal data, such as: name address, phone number, Social Security number, insurance company name, and insurance identification number. Include on the list the doctors and their numbers and a list of medications you are currently taking. You may want to add your immunizations that you had, and dates that you had them. If you have any allergies, if you are allergic to any medication, you should write it down also.

You may want to include your health proxy, your living will, and any instructions that you may have for your loved ones or your doctors in this file.

Let a family member or a friend know where you keep the medical file, in case it is needed and you are not in a condition to direct them to it.

Case # 10

Mrs. T. was not a client of our agency; she was a good friend of my parents. She was a widow, and quite independent, and in fairly good health up to the age of 83. I had been seeing her on all family gatherings, such as holiday dinners, birthdays, and other celebrations.

My mother called me one day to report that a hospital called her to notify her that her friend, Mrs. T. was taken to the hospital by ambulance after suffering a stroke. She was not able to give any personal information, but the nurse found my mother's phone number in her handbag, and called her.

I went to the hospital, and found my mother's friend in very serious condition. She survived the stroke, but there was a lot of damage done. Before bringing her home, I arranged for her home care aide, 24/7, through Medicaid, since she had no assets of her own.

While coordinating her medical treatment, I found out that for several years she had been suffering from high blood pressure, and had not followed doctors' orders; she had been taking medication at random, and there was also a question as to correct doses. This pattern caused her blood pressure to be very irregular, spiking to very dangerous levels, eventually causing her to have a massive stroke.

Now she is assisted by an aide who reminds her to take her medications on time and in the proper dose; Mrs. T. has a nurse visit weekly, who sorts her medication for the week; her blood pressure is controlled and the chance of another stroke is reduced.

While she was still in the hospital, I contacted Mrs. T's personal doctor, and we tried to figure out why she had not followed the instructions and taken her medications regularly. It became clear that she had not remembered the instructions, or remembered if she actually had taken the medication and at times took twice the dosage. This we realized when she finished her monthly supply a few days ahead of schedule.

To make matters more difficult, she had not coordinated her treatment between her family doctor and her cardiologist, and did not remember which medication was for which condition.

Since she functioned independently and no one checked her or followed up on her medical practices, for a long while she had managed to mask her forgetfulness and her early signs of confusion, putting her health in danger.

It took very little to establish a system where Ms T.'s doctors talked to each other and treatment was coordinated, with a nurse and an aide being involved.

At the time of this writing, she seems to be in fairly good health, with daily monitoring by her aide and a weekly visit from a nurse. I stop by weekly, checking with the support personnel, and making sure that all is well. We are all following her mental status, which is somewhat impaired, but with mental stimulation, the decline is not rapid and she seems to be happy, social, and well.

Chapter 6 –
Recognizing and Dealing with
Illnesses that Affect the Elderly

Dementia

There is a great deal of misunderstanding about dementia, not only by the layperson, but by professionals as well. From the view point of this book, I like to address the relation of dementia on the elderly, how it presents itself, and how it affects the one diagnosed with dementia and their family.

What is dementia?   Dementia is a progressive brain dysfunction that leads to a gradually increasing restriction of daily activities. The most well-known type of dementia is Alzheimer's disease. Dementia not only affects the patient, but also all the people surrounding them, and most patients who are diagnosed with dementia require care at different levels for the rest of their lives.

I am not a neurologist, and have not done any neurological studies, so I look at the different types of dementia from a lay perspective, basically in relation to the elderly, and describing in general strokes some of the conditions that can affect the elderly in the later years.

From the data available today we surmise the following:

Some disorders that cause progressive deterioration in any part of one's nervous system can produce a collection of signs and symptoms (syndrome) called dementia.

Dementia is characterized by a progressive decline in intellectual and social abilities, to a degree that interferes with daily functioning. Not all patients experience the same symptoms, and most of them vary from individual to individual. In each individual suffering from dementia signs and symptoms depend on their genetic make-up, lifestyle, cultural background, and personal life experiences. In general, one can say that in most dementia patients the symptoms that present themselves are: memory loss, deficits in judgment and language, as well as in reasoning. And as dementia progresses, changes in personality and abnormal behavior may also present themselves. Eventually, dementia patients may lose the ability to perform the most basic tasks, and the ability to communicate with their environment.

As of today, there is no known cure for degenerative brain disorders, but science is progressing. In the last decade, we learned more about the brain than was known about it in the last 100 years. Neurological science has become a desirable area of study in colleges across the country. My own daughter, Danielle, chose it as her major, and the study of the brain holds for her a great fascination.

Thus, it is possible that in the near future we will make strides in understanding the mechanics of the brain, and find preventive methods, and cures for brain degeneration.

For now, a few of the diseases of the brain that can bring on dementia are:

Alzheimer's Disease

Alzheimer's disease is the most common cause of dementia. The changes that manifest themselves in people with Alzheimer's include a loss of nerve cells in the vital areas to memory and other mental functions. Patients with Alzheimer's have lower levels of brain chemicals that carry messages back and forth between nerve cells. As mentioned in the Alzheimer's section in this book, the signs for the disease are: forgetfulness, language, reasoning, and comprehension deficiencies, as well as reading and writing difficulties. In later stages, anxiousness and aggressive behavior may present themselves as well.

Parkinson's Disease

Parkinson's disease was first described by James Parkinson in England in 1817. It is a progressive degeneration of nerve cells (neurons) in parts of the brain that control muscle movements.

Parkinson's disease manifests itself in various ways. It may be evident on one side or both sides of the body. We blink, smile, swing our arms when we walk, and all those are unconscious acts of human behavior. In Parkinson's patients this acts tend to be lost. Many will develop a fixed staring expression and unblinking eyes: the so called-masked face.

During the later stages of the disease, as many as 30 to 40 percent of people with Parkinson's disease develop dementia, with the loss of intellectual and social abilities.

Vascular Dementia

Vascular dementia results either from narrowing and blockage of the arteries that supply blood flow to the brain, or from strokes that result from an interruption of blood flow to the brain. The onset of symptoms is often abrupt, but at times the disease may progress slowly, making it difficult to distinguish it from Alzheimer's disease. With this condition, it is common to experience problems with thinking, language, walking, bladder control, and vision.

Front Temporal Dementia

Front temporal dementia is an uncommon brain disorder characterized by disturbance in behavior, personality and eventually memory. The disease is relentless in its progression and may ultimately include language impairment, erratic behavior and, dementia. Pick's disease is a form of front temporal dementia.

Creutzfeldt-Jakob Disease

Dementia that sometimes occurs in young or middle-aged people may be caused by Creutzfeldt-Jakob disease. This rare and fatal brain disorder is thought to be caused by prions, infectious agents that can transform normal protein molecules into transmissible, deadly ones.

The earliest signs and symptoms of the disease may be memory impairment and behavior changes. The disease progresses rapidly with mental deterioration, muscle jerks (involuntary movements), weakness of the limbs, blindness, and eventually coma.

Huntington's Disease

Huntington's disease stems from an inherited disorder within the brain that causes certain nerve cells in the brain to waste away. As the disorder progresses, patient experience personality changes, and a decline in intellect, memory, speech and judgment. Dementia may develop in the later stages of the disease.

Disorders that mimic dementia:

Some conditions produce signs and symptoms similar to those of dementia, particularly in older adults. Two conditions sometimes mistaken for dementia are depression and delirium.

Depression can cause difficulty in remembering, thinking clearly, and concentrating. Sometimes, depression occurs in conjunction with dementia. In those cases, the deterioration of emotions and intellect can be more extreme.

Delirium is an acute state in temporary mental confusion. It tends to be most common in older adults who have lung or heart disease, infections, poor nutrition, medication reactions, or hormone disorders. A person who exhibits sudden disorientation, loss of mental skills, or loss of consciousness is likely to have delirium rather than dementia.

The above descriptions are very basic and limited, and their intent is to give you a general overview of different symptoms and causes of dementia. There is extensive and more in-depth material on the subject that can be found in print and on the Internet. Patients exhibiting any of the above-mentioned symptoms should be directed to a neurologist for evaluation, diagnosis and care.

The Different Stages of Dementia and Its effects on Family and Patient.

1. The first stage tends to be the hardest for the patient. He or she may understand and recognize that something is wrong, and try to mask it.

2. The second stage is the hardest for the caregiver. In this stage the patient may be the most uncooperative, and difficult to take care of.

3. The third stage is the hardest for the primary decision-maker. This stage tends to be very emotionally taxing for the decision-maker regarding the patient, especially if he or she is related to the patient and knew them at better times of life.

Initial Stage:

This period lasts on the average up to four years. The following changes may be noted:

1. Persistent short memory loss.
2. May be able to mask lapses of memory in initial stages.
3. May be social and alert, but knows something is wrong.
4. Poor concentration and difficulty retaining new information.
5. Forgets appointments, dates, and names.
6. Puts things in wrong places, leaves stove on.
7. May forget to pay a bill, or pay it twice.
8. May be susceptible to money scams.
9. May begin to withdraw from social activities.
10. May get lost when driving.
11. Repeats stories, or questions.
12. Has problems naming common objects.
13. May display moodiness and/or hostility.
14. Personal hygiene can start slipping.
15. Refuses help at home.
16. May decide that he/she does not need medication, and stop taking it.
17. May be easily upset or depressed.

Next Stage:

The middle period tend to be the longest of the three periods, it may last up to 10 years. The following are some of the changes that can be noted in the patient's behavior:

1. Increased memory loss, and decreased attention span.
2. Increased impaired judgment.
3. Repeats himself in a short time span.

4. Progresses to bigger accidents, while driving the car.

5. Decrease of care in personal appearance.

6. May get lost in familiar places.

7. Increased suspicion in people surrounding them and the environment in general.

8. Decreased appetite.

9. Refuses help with ADL's (activities of daily living).

10. May start to wander around with no purpose.

11. May lose personal items and then think they were stolen.

12. May hear and see things that are not there.

13. May become hostile, aggressive, and uncooperative.

14. Sleeping patterns change, may nap during the day, and wander during the night.

15. May repeat meaningless tasks, with greater frequency.

16. May not recognize people outside his or her immediate circle.

17. Beginning to experience urinary incontinence.

18. Spends more time in bed.

19. Becomes restless in the afternoon. As dementia progresses, long-term memory begins to fail.

Final Stage:

In this stage the patient tends to require total care, and in all likelihood is totally depended on others for care. This is the shortest period, lasting about three years.

1. Disorientation to time and place.

2. May not recognize relatives, caretakers, and possibly him or herself in the mirror.

3. Requires 24-hour care.

4. May lose weight, even while eating well.

5. Exhibits difficulties to swallow, possibly will need to be fed.

6. Will become totally incontinent.

7. Unable to get out of bed or chair without assistance.

8. Becomes non-communicative, speaking in unrelated sentences. Or not speaking at all.

9. At the end of this stage, the patient will be totally bedridden, and mostly sleeping.

10. Will become susceptible to malnutrition, infections, and pneumonia.

Dementia and Communication

People with dementia usually have problems with communication. Their use of language and understanding others is impaired. The most common changes that are noticeable in dementia patients in fairly early stages are repetition and the use of inaccurate and socially inappropriate words that may reflect jealousy, paranoia, or impulsiveness.

The following are some guidelines to help you communicate with a person who has dementia:

1. Approach the person from the front, identify yourself, and address the patient by name.

2. Speak slowly and clearly, in a gentle and relaxed voice.

3. Use short, simple, and familiar words. Repeat when necessary, using the same word.

4. Use one-steps commands and requests.

5. Ask one question at a time, preferably those that can be answered with a yes or no.

6. Give the person extra time to respond.

7. Offer encouragement when the person is having difficulties expressing themselves.

8. Do not interrupt, criticize, correct, or argue.

9. Be patient and flexible.

10. Identify people by name.

11. Avoid negative statements and quizzing, such as "you know who that is, don't you?"

12. Let the person know that you are listening and trying to understand.

13. Maintain eye contact, to show interest.

14. Do not talk about the patient to others, as if they are not there.

15. Use non-verbal communication, such pointing and touching, when it is appropriate.

16. Provide appropriate touch. This perhaps is the greatest form of communication in the advanced stages of dementia. Offering hugs, applying hand lotion and giving back rubs can be wonderful ways to communicate to the patient that you care, and accept them, as they are.

The above chapter was written to provide you with the tools to identify early stages of dementia and to be able to step in and seek out appropriate professional help to assist the patient by providing care. I am focusing more extensively on the subject of dementia due to the underlying implications that present themselves with the appearance of symptoms.

Initially, the symptoms may be masked by the patient, in an effort to fool the people around them from recognizing the mental changes that are occurring. But it is very important that the people around such patients be alert and attuned to the changes, and steps in as soon as possible to mitigate the symptoms and slow them down with medical intervention, if possible, and prevent any harm that may occur as a result.

We should also understand that if someone close to us becomes afflicted with dementia, it is not only their behavior that will change, but we, too, will change. We will need to adapt a new pattern of behavior in relation to them, to become more attuned to their needs and mental and physical abilities.

Case # 11

One of our first patients with dementia was a lady in her late 80s. Ms. K. had never married and had lived all her life with her mother and father, until their deaths, a few months apart, in 1973. When our agency stepped in to take care of Ms. K. with 24-hour service, she apparently had been confused for a while and it was sheer luck that she had not done harm to herself or the residents in her apartment building.

Ms. K. continued to live in the same apartment, without throwing out anything at all. When we began to provide services, it was impossible to cross the living room or enter the bedrooms. The bedrooms were stocked with boxes of clothing, old newspapers, empty and full boxes of food products, mail that had never been opened, etc.

It is not that unusual to see an apartment of an elderly person that is over-cluttered with items no longer used. Ms. K.'s apartment was far beyond that. I do not know how she managed to live there for so many years, without it burning down, although apparently she came close to just that.

The apartment had not been painted for at least forty years; chunks of plaster hung from the ceilings, and fell from the wall, where it was visible above the trash and boxes. Ms. K. kept every detergent containers, every cleaning can, after she used up their contents, as well as jars and plastic containers from sour cream or cottage cheese, that were not washed out.

The smell was unbearable inside the apartment and in the hallway. This, apparently, caused the neighbors to call the protective services to step in and evaluate Ms. K. They were able to find her doctor's information and, although she had not seen him for at least ten years, he remembered her and offered to contact us.

The hardest issue we had to deal with while providing home care for Ms. K. was to make her living space safe for her, physically and health-wise. It was not easy; she refused to have anything at all thrown out. We had no choice, but to throw out boxes and suitcases full of trash that she picked up through the years off the street discarded by others. This was done when she slept on the sofa in the living room. She could not sleep in the bedroom as the bed was piled up with trash on top of it, and around it.

Ms K kept saying that her mother did not allow the removal of any-thing in the apartment, she needed it all. But as the apartment was cleared of more and more trash, she did not seem to miss it, or even be aware that the clutter was being slowly reduced.

Broken pieces of furniture were removed and eventually we could arrange for Ms. K. to actually sleep in a bed. With the cooperation of the landlord, her apartment was painted. The rotten carpet was pulled up, and the wooden floor was polished, and turned out to be beautiful.

Although Ms. K.'s confusion increased, with care and the safe environment, she lived to be 95 years old, and until the day she died, continued to live in her home safely.

Alzheimer's-The big Misconception

Alzheimer's is turning to be one of the epidemics of the 21st century. Currently, about 4.5 million Americans are diagnosed with different stages of Alzheimer's. Their diagnosis affects millions of other Americans, their relatives, friends and caregivers. It also affects the taxpayer, for the burden of cost is great.

Initial diagnosis is made usually when the disease manifests itself in a fairly obvious way. The average age of a person who is diagnosed with Alzheimer's is around 85 years.

It is projected that close to 50% of all elderly will display some form of dementia. The age factor seems to be the single greatest risk for Alzheimer's. Although Alzheimer's has been recognized for more than 30 years, there is still a lack of understanding of the disease by the public at large, and to some degree by medical and clinical providers. Most geriatric teams are trained in diagnosis, but the actual caregivers are not trained in specific needs of care for the Alzheimer's patient.

Alzheimer's is a progressive and a debilitating disease. As better and more accurate techniques of diagnosis are developed, and more effective medications are developed and made available, care and management of the disease will improve.

Alzheimer's disease gradually robs a person of the ability to remember, reason, and make decisions in the most basic daily life tasks.

The National Institute on Aging (NIA), reports that after the age of 65, the prevalence of Alzheimer's cases doubles every five years.

Due to the fact that the baby boomers are entering this age group in very high numbers, it is projected that the diagnosed cases of Alzheimer's will spike accordingly.

The Alzheimer's Foundation of America (AFA) projects the number of Alzheimer's cases will triple in the next 50 years. That's about 15 million patients suffering from this debilitating illness. The impact of this on our society in cost and cultural effects will be enormous. It is estimated that Alzheimer's will cost Medicare about $400 billion in 25 years. That's more than the entire Medicare budget currently.

By delaying the onset of Alzheimer's, we can reduce the health care cost for people with the disease by 50%. Even delaying the institutionalizing of Alzheimer's patients in nursing homes by one month will save $1 billion annually.

As of today, no one knows what causes this disease, but certain risks factors have been identified. The risk of developing Alzheimer's in later years rises, although it is not part of the normal aging process. Due to predisposition, or genetic factors, Alzheimer's seems also to run in families, especially if there is a member in the family that had an early onset of the disease.

Memory loss is usually the first sign to signal some changes. All of us tend to exhibit some memory loss, which is normal. We usually remember recent events; but with Alzheimer's, short-term memory is lost. Other symptoms include pronounced absentmindedness and a visible inability to concentrate.

As the disease progresses, the symptoms become more obvious. It becomes not only the failure of remember, but also to understand what has happened. If the patient did not remember the word "telephone" before, now he or she will not know what to do with the phone when it rings.

This makes functioning very difficult for the person, and when patient reaches this stage, he or she can not be on their own. The common public impression of Alzheimer's and other dementias is that they are characterized by a slow, quiet slide into permanent helplessness and memory loss. In fact, the slide is very rapid in many cases, and it is not a gentle fade into the blackness. Care should be provided, or an appropriate residential facility should be found.

It is estimated that 87 percent of Alzheimer's patients are cared for by relatives. The toll is high in terms of manpower lost in the economic market. And the emotional toll is immeasurable.

To find your loved one in this kind situation may be most alarming, and you need to become educated regarding the different stages of this disease. Among the changes that occur are also personality changes. At times you may have difficulties to see the friendly and social person that you have known all your life. They may have mood swings, from happy to sad, from calm to tears and anger. And you will not know what set it off, because there need not be a reason at all.

The inevitable cognitive and physical decline of the Alzheimer's patient takes a toll on the caregiver and the family. It is an emotionally wrenching and physically exhausting responsibility. Alzheimer's is a progressive, irreversible brain disease, in which metabolism and chemistry in the nerve cell falter. To put plainly: the cell dies.

With today's state of the art neurological and laboratory tests, a doctor with dementia experience can make an accurate diagnosis before the patient dies. Part of the diagnosis is to assess the patient's sense of place and time, simple exercises to test memory level, as well as simple math problems. Level of retention is looked at. At times, neurologists will order an MRI of the brain to eliminate any possibility of brain tumors.

According to the NIA, Alzheimer's may be long in duration from two to twenty years, but in majority of cases, the Alzheimer's patient will live between eight and ten years.

There are some drugs currently available, and with the continued research, more improved versions will find their way to the market, which will help to slow down the progression of this disease. In addition to a regimen of medication, memory exercises should be provided for the person, such as a list of daily activities, simple instructions, labeling items that the patient uses daily, and constant verbal reinforcement.

Research suggests that currently, diagnosis of an Alzheimer's patient is usually delayed by two years. As we know, although dementia is a physical illness, it manifests itself in behavioral patterns. To establish a list of guidelines, to help you recognize the early stages of Alzheimer's, the following signs may be helpful:

a. Short term memory loss

b. Difficulties retaining new information

c. Lost or misplaced objects

d. Neglecting household chores

e. Poor personal hygiene

f. Careless appearance

g. Unsafe decisions

h. Decrease in language skills

i. Decreased interest in previous hobbies

j. Decrease in social interaction

k. Decrease interest in family and friends

l. Changes in old habits

If you recognize patterns of behavior from the above list in your parent, you have to take action. Your parent or parents cannot be left to their own device, and most decision-making should be shifted to the person that will centralize all issues touching their everyday life. There should be an emergency plan of action in place prior to an actual emergency occurring. (95% of all inquires regarding long term care are due to some medical emergency). See the chapter dealing with emergency planning.

As of today, we do not know how to prevent this disease from happening, nor do we know how to stop it when it does happen. But from the research to date, it seems that there is some benefit in providing mental stimulation, visual mental exercises, and good nutrition. Most importantly, make sure that appropriate medical care is provided, and the patient sees a neurologist who specializes in dementia.

With the realization of how widespread this problem is, there are more and more funds available for research. Hopefully, in the not so distant future, scientists will develop either a preventive medication, such as a vaccination, or a therapeutic medication that will slow the advancement of this devastating disease.

Case # 12

My aunt was diagnosed with Alzheimer's some years ago. It did not come as a shock to us, but we tried to fool ourselves for quite a few years before the diagnosis came. She is a Holocaust survivor, and like my parents, lived through a hellish nightmare during World War II and survived. Her life, as with the rest of the survivors, was not easy, but she built her existence with courage and not a drop of resentment as to the hand that life had dealt her.

She married, but was unable to have children, and worked hard as a menial worker, as she didn't have the luxury of benefiting from higher education or any vocational training. In those days one struggled to provide food and clothing for herself and her husband, there was no time for training.

In her early 70s she lost her husband, who suffered from Parkinson's for many years. During all the years that she took care of her husband, all our attention was directed toward him. We all were worried about him, and followed the stages of his illness. None of us paid much attention to the telltale signs that were becoming more and more pronounced in her behavior. Being as intelligent as she was, and maybe sensing that something was wrong with her, she hid a lot of signs.

She also compensated in very brave ways to make her confusion not as easily detectable. She began to stumble while speaking, searching for words, stopping in mid sentence, hesitating, using wrong words that were similar, but different than the meaning she was trying to get across.

She used humor to cover the shortcomings. Yet when visiting her and spending more time with her than I usually did in a short phone conversation, I started to be aware of the change in the pattern of her speech. I began to realize that she, too, was aware of the situation, and was trying even harder to compensate for it. I alerted her personal physician, suggesting that maybe some evaluations should be done and precautionary measures should be put in place.

She fought us tooth and nail; "I am okay, just forgetting some things, and it is natural for people my age" she would say. It took some time to establish a safe environment which followed a good plan (the one outlined in the chapter on safety).

Even with some medical intervention, her condition had progressed rapidly. She began to wander in the neighborhood, left empty pots on a lit stove, and it's only by God's mercy that her house did not go up in flames.

My aunt was always involved in her community, volunteering, or partaking in social activities in the local center for senior citizens. She always loved art, sewing, and embroidering, and her work was displayed at the center.

When she became cognizant of her failing memory, forgetting the names of the others in the center and forgetting what she should do with her project midway through it, she began to feel very uncomfortable, and refused to continue attending. This was very disconcerting to all of us, because she became reclusive, anti-social, and depressed.

She also started to lose weight. It was time to step in. With the help of a local agency, we brought in a home aide for eight hours a day, on the weekends relatives rotated the responsibilities of her care. We found a different senior center, with a program that was geared for people with Alzheimer's. She did not know the people there, which made it easier for her; she did not have to justify the fact that she did not remember their names.

Many of the activities were subtle: exercises in memory rejuvenation and establishing tools and tricks to help the participants to remember and function in the best of their ability in spite of the illness that was robbing them of their memories. Specialists in the treatment of people with Alzheimer's provided much needed help and guidance to make the home geared to promote normalization and a sense of familiarity.`

When we visit with my aunt, we introduce ourselves by name, to eliminate the need for her to guess who the person in front of her is. The key is to make her life safe, comfortable, and full of love, which she had always bestowed in great amounts on all of us when she could.

There are about 4,000 adult day care centers currently operating in the United States They provide a social environment and there are meals served in them to the people attending, and many provide other services, such as a social worker, nurses, and information regarding home care services.

Most of these day care centers provide recreational programs and even trips. Approximately half of the seniors benefiting from these centers are diagnosed with Alzheimer's. Most of the participants also have other medical problems that may or may not complicate the problems stemming from their Alzheimer's.

The day care centers also, in most cases, are equipped to care for the disabled and the frail, in their daily programs. They also provide transportation, picking the seniors up from their homes and dropping them off at the end of the day. This makes it so much easier for the family, and relieves much stress from their day, worrying about their loved ones wellbeing and safety.

Search the neighborhood for a center that can provide the services you will need for your parent or loved one. The proximity to the center is secondary to the services they provide. Especially if they provide transportation, the distance will be less of problem. To help you find such a program in your state, check the section for Alzheimer's Association contacts on our site: www.goldenyearsgolden.com .

It is hard to watch our parent or a loved one struggling with Alzheimer's especially as they worsen through each stage. Each stage presents different sets of problems, which affect each individual differently. There is a lot of research being done at this time, and we are likely to eventually see new techniques and more accurate diagnosis, as well as better treatment. Who knows? Maybe the baby boomers will be the beneficiaries of these future breakthroughs.

Chronic Illnesses

One of the realizations that the medical community has come to terms with is that as people live longer, they will develop more chronic diseases. Although not all chronic diseases can be cured, the level of severeness and the impact of symptoms on the patient's everyday life can be reduced, and perhaps minimized with education, prevention, and proper care.

Maintaining your health as long as possible should be a life-long goal. Some chronic illnesses can be prevented, or their onset pushed back. One of the things that you can do to improve your ability to maintain a good life is to be physically active.

One can be physically active during any period in one's life, and at any stage of a chronic illness – or at least to the level that one is able. The elderly tend to become sedentary, and in most cases, this exacerbates their chronic illness symptoms. When starting any physical activity regiment make sure to clear it with your doctor first, starting slowly, and increasing the rate gradually.

Regular medical examinations should be part of the life of the elderly, not to mention the entire population as it ages. Medicare provides us with free medical examinations after the age of 60, when we are eligible to join their system. But its program, as of now has limitations and restrictions.

Although chronic diseases, such as heart disease, diabetes, and obesity, have become fairly common, our health system and our caregivers, continue to concentrate on acute treatment and episodic treatment, rather than preventive and long-term treatment.

Frequently, patients with chronic illnesses have more than one illness, suffering from multiple problems with overlapping symptoms, complicating treatment and increasing the severity of the illness.

Chronic illnesses may complicate a person's life by increasing their dependency on others for daily care, such as assistance in daily activities, bathing, and dressing, shopping, cleaning, and cooking.

Without such help, they may not be able to keep doctor appointments, maintain a stable regimen of prescription drug use, and avoid flare-ups of their chronic illness that may be avoidable.

Any revamping of the health care system needs to take this into account and develop support systems to aid the chronically ill. If the patient ends up needing to use emergency care in the hospital, because he had not accessed preventive care or maintained a regular visiting pattern with his doctors, it increases the cost of treatments by a great deal. That ends up to be a burden to the taxpayer.

The pharmaceutical treatment of chronic diseases has to become much more controlled. Considering that a chronically ill person has to take medication to treat his or her condition - for the duration of their life in most cases - it has to be possible for them to pay for that medication.

As of now many people who are uninsured, or who do not qualify for Medicare part D, or who are in the $2,000 to $3,500 range, which part D will not cover, are unable to afford the medication. In those cases, the condition deteriorates without the treatment of the prescribed medication, increasing the severity of the condition, shortening the life of the patient, or causing unnecessary pain and suffering.

In general, pharmaceutical costs have to be reduced for all Americans. If we cannot afford the medication, what good can these medical science breakthroughs be to us? It seems that the drugs remain prohibitively expensive in the United States, and yet we are subsidizing lower cost for the same medications in other countries. I do believe that we should help countries in need, but it should be prioritized: we owe it to our citizens to provide them with an accessible health care system and attainable medication when needed.

To cut costs we should encourage generic drug use. Until drugs are available at reasonable prices, people should be encouraged to purchase in groups, where negotiations can be made to purchase drugs at the best possible prices.

Educational programs should be made available to teach the general population how to purchase medications in the most cost-efficient way, and to use medications safely and wisely.

We should import prescription medication from other countries, such as Canada, to reduce cost of medication, with the provision that the medication is safe and meets the standards of our FDA.

Chapter 7 –
Providing Care- Do Your Homework

Safety for the Elderly

The biggest danger to our elders and their health is an unsafe environment. It is well known that, for seniors, falls are the worst things that can happen to them; many seniors do not recover completely from them. Fractures can put them in a wheelchair, and render them non-ambulatory for the rest of their lives. The healing process can be lengthy and complicated by other conditions that they may suffer from, such as diabetes, a poor immune system, etc.

In this chapter I will address personal safety of the elderly in their residential environment. I will touch on the general environment in the society at large, pointing out existing safety measures, and those that should be developed and put into place.

Before getting into the safety of the physical environment, and how to make it as safe as possible, I am compelled to stress again the need to always be on the lookout for tell-tale signs of mental and physical abuse. That is where the need begins.

When visiting an elderly person, ill, or dependent on others, always be alert to the following signs:

a. Emotional or Psychological Abuse:
   Are there insults or threats directed at the elder? Are they living in social isolation? The person may be extremely upset, withdrawn, unresponsive, or exhibiting other unusual behavior. He or she may have a vacant look in their eyes or exhibit fear; they may not always express those verbally, so look for signs in their face or behavior.

b. Physical and Sexual Abuse:
   Look for suspicious bruises or other injuries. Look for signs of restraints, such as a rope burns. See if he or she shows sudden changes in behavior, such as unexplained anger, withdrawal, or becoming very quiet. Note if a worker or caregiver refuses to let you visit the elder, making all kind of excuses.

c. Neglect:
   Look for signs of malnutrition, if there is noticeable weight loss, dehydration, bed sores, or if personal hygiene is noticeably neglected. Note if the elder is in soiled clothing, unkempt, without dentures, with long nails or dirty nails, unshaven, or at midday walking around in night clothing. Listen to complaints the elder voices, if she or he complains about the aide not listening to them or disregarding their wishes and instructions. You should follow up on their complaint with the personal aide, because it may lead to discovery of abuse and neglect.

d. Financial Abuse:
   If you notice unexplained bank withdrawals, unauthorized use of bank and credit cards, as well as reports of stolen or missing checkbooks and bank cards, or if your parent or elder writes checks as a loan or gift to the aide. Keep an eye out for sudden changes in the will or banking documents, these trigger a red alert. Be alert if assets are suddenly transferred to a family member or to someone outside the family, valuables suddenly disappear, the elder suddenly makes unwise investments, or a distant relative suddenly appears to claim the right to handle the finances.

If you become aware of any of the above warning signals, you should correct them, and/or notify the police. The above warning signs should be looked for not only at the home of the elderly, but also if he or she resides in a nursing home, a residential care facility, or an assisted living facility.

Preparing the Home or Apartment for Emergency Needs

While evaluating the present situation of your loved one for changes or improvements, you have to prepare for times of emergency.

As your parent ages, and his or her physical needs change, you should take a walk through their home to make sure that they are safe there.

1. Start with the bathroom. Most accidents happen there. Make sure that there are safety bars in the bathtub or shower. Put a shower chair in the bathtub or shower. If it is possible to build a stall shower, to be used instead of the bathtub, it makes it easier for the elderly person to get in and out of the shower. Make sure to have a low step into the shower. Make sure that hot water faucets are a safe distance from the body. Make sure that the floor is not slippery, by perhaps covering it with a rug that is heavy and will not be easily moved. Make sure that toiletries can be easily reached and not placed too high. A safety and support bar should be near the toilet to help the elderly to sit down and to stand up from the toilet. If possible, install reversible hinges on the bathroom door, making it easy to push out the door while maneuvering a wheelchair, if ever needed. Make sure that there is a bell or emergency phone in the bathroom in a reachable position.

2. In the kitchen, products and dishes, cups and such, must be easy to reach for your loved one, so that there is no need for the everyday use of ladders and stools. Lighting for the stove and for the use of small appliances should be adequate. Place a smoke alarm and fire extinguisher in the kitchen. When purchasing food supplies, select boxes and canned goods that are easy for the elderly to open. You will find a great deal of gadgets that are helpful for this task. Check weekly as to the status of food supplies in your loved one's house. Keep select foods that do not require refrigeration, such as some canned food, soups and vegetables, and cookies, pasta, crackers, coffee, and sugar if they use it. Also important are powdered milk, dried fruits, protein bars, and a few cans of nutritional supplements. Make sure that you keep a few gallons of bottled water for emergencies.

3. In the living room, make sure that all electric plugs work, and no loose electrical wires are exposed or are in spots that can cause tripping. Make a place for the remote control, such as a plastic shoe box; this way the remote will not fall constantly, and your parent will not have to look for it under the furniture. It is beneficial for your

parent to have furniture that allows for comfortable sitting, and if the sofa or chairs are slightly higher, it will make it easier for them to get up from a sitting position without assistance. Periodically, check all chairs in the house for safety, to make sure that they are sturdy and are not easily turned over. Wall-to-wall carpeting is the safest flooring; avoid area rugs, which can slide or cause tripping; tile or wood floors can be slippery when wet.

4. In the bedroom, again, make sure that there is an emergency bell and/ or phone. Encourage a routine where your parent brings in a glass of water for the night, discouraging night trips for a drink. Make sure that your parent has some form of support in getting into and out of bed, i.e. something to lean on or hold onto. Have an extra blanket within reach. If eventually there is a need, it may be a good idea to order a commode that will decrease the trips to the bathroom during the night, thus decreasing the potential for accidents. Always have a nightlight in the room and in the hallway. A motion-sensitive bulb that automatically illuminates in the dark is ideal so that the elderly person doesn't have to remember to turn the light on.

5. Medication: Organize the medication in a way to decrease confusion. A weekly medication box can be filled, with the medication set up by the days, and specific times of the day, such as morning, noon, afternoon, and evening. You will find below some suggestions as to different medication boxes, some of which are very sophisticated. This will help guard against forgetfulness, and make it easy to see if indeed the medications were taken at the right time. On a board or a refrigerator, in large letters and numbers, post emergency numbers of the doctors who care for your loved one, numbers of the nearest hospital, and the pharmacy they use. The insurance information, such as the I.D. number and phone number, should also be placed there. Medicare and Medicaid numbers should be included, as well, to have them handy.

On the market today are several medication organizers. Some are:

- MED-CENTER, a talking pillbox. It costs around $70, it organizes a month's worth of medication, and the pillbox alerts you to take your medication four times a day. If you want more information from this company, call 1-866-600-3244, or go to www.medcentersystems.com.

- MULTI ALARM PILL BOX & EASY SET TIMER. This device allows you to set up more than 30 alarms; it not only tells you when to take the dose, it reports back to the caretaker. This device costs about $49.

- RESCUE ALERT monitors the pill box directly. The pill box has a transmitter implanted in the box which will activate if the pill box was not opened within 15 or 30 minutes of the scheduled medication time. There are a few plans either to rent or outright purchase. To find out details and cost, call 1-800-688-9576, or go to www.rescuealert.com.

6. Personal hygiene items to make sure you have: Toothpaste and toothbrush, toilet paper and paper towels, garbage bags, soap, shampoo, and cleaning supplies.

7. First Aid Kit: Rubber gloves, antibiotic cream and burn ointment are musts. Cold packs; adhesive bandages, cotton balls, swabs, sterile dressing, tape, and elastic wrap, a thermometer, sharp scissors, eyewash solution, medication for fever and pain relief, such as acetaminophen or ibuprofen, and antihistamines are also necessary. If your loved one takes medication on a regular basis, extra should be stored here in the event that access to a pharmacy is impossible in an emergency.

8. Tools: Manual can opener, flashlight, battery-powered light sticks, portable battery-powered radio, batteries, matches, duct tape, wrench or pliers.

9. Additional items: Spare eyeglasses and hearing aid batteries.
   Copies of credit cards, bank account numbers, copies of important documents, a list of medications being taken, a copy of the driver's license and passport, a copy of the insurance card, Medicare card, Medicaid card, Social Security card, and birth certificate. Keys should be kept handy and an extra set of keys left with someone nearby, such as a neighbor or a friend.

10. Cell phone for the parent. Keep a list of phone numbers of doctors, the nearest hospital, and nearest pharmacy. List numbers that your

parent can call in time of need. Keep a copy of the same lists of numbers at your home, so you have them handy in case you need to make a call, or if your parent has misplaced his or her documents.

11. If possible, install lever-type handles on the doors in the apartment or house, to make opening the doors easy for people who may suffer from arthritis or are generally weak. The grip of such handles is easy and steady.

12. If the apartment or house in which your parent lives has stairs, indoor or outdoor, make sure that both sides of the stairs have railings.

13. A bench or a chair in front of their main entrance door will help them to rest, or to put their bags down, while they find their keys. When you think about it, we can all use a bench in front of our entry doors, and it can be a decorative piece as well.

Among the steps that you take to provide a safe environment for your loved one, you should consider providing them with an SOS button. There are quite a few devices on the market, and you can pick the most suitable one for you. They are essentially a wireless hotline to seek help. Considering that a third of elderly people live on their own, the device may be a lifesaver for them.

Some of the more popular brands are:

- PHILIPS LIFELINE: The initial payment costs you $75, and then $1 per day for the monitoring. Contact 1-800-543-3546 or www.lifelinesys.com.

- RESCUE ALERT: This device can be either bought or rented. The initial fee is $29. Contact: 1-800-688-9576, or www.rescuealert.com.

- ADT COMPANION SERVICE: This device costs $99 to set up, and a monthly fee of $35. Contact: 1-800-209-7599, or www.adt.com.

- READY RESPONSE: The cost is $35 initially for the set-up, with a monthly fee of $35. Contact: 1-866-310-9061, or www. walgreens.com.

There are many other help-call devices, in addition to the ones that are mentioned above. I do not particularly recommend one over another; pick whichever is the right one for you.

Truly, the list is useful for all of us, but we usually don't think that we need those items "right now." But we all do. So while taking care of putting together your parent's emergency needs, do yourself a favor and put together your own.

The above precautions and considerations refer to the home of your loved one. But you should apply the safety evaluation for any place the elder spends time. If your parent has outside grounds that he or she uses, check those too for any possible accident promoters, such as loose steps, rocks, etc.

If your parent lives in a residential care facility, in a shared housing situation, in a retirement community, all of the above apply.

If your parent is in a nursing home, or any other long-term care facility, check his or her room for safety. Walk through the common rooms to see if there are any items on the floor that could cause tripping such as loose electric cords or any other cables. Also check the bathrooms for safety bars.

Visit the facility at meal times to see if the food is served safely, and if there are a sufficient number of personnel overseeing the dining room. Are there enough aides to feed the patients that need to be fed? In the years that I worked in nursing homes, I found that too few aides were responsible for the dining areas, which translated into patients being rushed during feeding, and not always being given proper attention. This brings up the question of whether the patients are intaking the appropriate amount of nutrition. If you see many very skinny residents, it may be due to inadequate nutrition.

If your parent needs to be fed, or encouraged to eat, this is extremely important. An insufficient number of personnel could promote poor intake of food, due to rushed or incomplete feedings, and before long you will see your parent losing weight. Poor eating may cause deficiencies, weakness, poor health, and decreased mental alertness.

Although it may seem odd to include feeding in the safety chapter, it is definitely a safety issue for the patient, since poor nutrition will reflect on their overall health. I will also discuss feeding in the chapter dealing with nutrition, as well as in the chapter on choosing the right nursing home.

Case # 13

Very early in our agency's existence, when we did not yet have many patients, I was able to spend a great deal of personal time with each patient. Thus when Ms. D. needed home care, I met her personally and was quite impressed with her vitality and independence.

Truly I did not know if she actually needed assistance at that particular junction in her life. Her daughters, both living in another state, hours away from their mother, insisted that she begin home care in order to decrease the chances of accidents and problems.

Ms. D. was very pleasant and social, and quite polite to the aides, but refused any help and assistance offered to her. She was very resentful that this assistance was forced upon her by her daughters, and she was paying for it from her own savings.

As a rule, I do not like to get between the senior and their family, but the daughters were insistent. I had a feeling the daughters knew more than they were telling us. It is essential that we know all the relevant information about the patient so that we can provide them with the best care possible. Something about this situation just did not feel right.

I visited Ms. D. a few times, establishing a friendly bond, and she kept maintaining her opinion that she did not need an aide. The aides literally spent their eight hours with her sitting and reading, because she refused to let them do any work at all.

I explained to Ms. D.'s daughters that if this continued, we would have to discontinue services. Just then they told me that their mother had tried to take her life twice and suffered from depression, and they feared that she would try again; that is why they forced home care services on her.

Knowing the underlying problem, we could then develop a good care plan for the patient. We placed an older woman with Ms. D. and we asked if the daughters could pay for the services at least initially, in order to reduce resentment on their mother's part and the fear that she would deplete her savings.

Things improved fairly quickly from then on. Ms. D. developed a very stable and friendly relationship with her aide, and slowly started to share responsibility for the household chores. They did social activities together, and became more like friends than patient and worker.

In addition, Ms. D. visited her doctors regularly, for her physical as well as mental health. We were there for her when the lows set in, and kept her safe, recognizing the signs, and making sure her doctors knew when a crisis was looming.

It felt good to make sure that Ms. D. was well, living her life safely and to the fullest.

First Stage Help-The Case Manager

In recent years a new profession has developed called the case manager. As the population is aging and children are living far from their parents, in many cases, a need developed. That's where the case manager comes in. We have case managers in social services, in educational services, in military services, and in medical services for many years. So, in the last few years, we have started to see case managers stepping in to help the elderly and their families.

In the private sector, these case managers are for the most part educated in social services and geriatrics. Some have experience in nursing homes and hospitals, but there are many who do not have formal education in related areas to benefit the elderly, and are basically administrators. It is up to you to check their background, and their credentials.

The case manager will take on the responsibility of coordinating the care of the elderly, including:

1. Assess the elderly for the care she or he may require.

2. Determines if the elderly is eligible for different services.

3. Is the contact point for all the relevant agencies or individuals to process the required documentation.

4. Interviews, hires, and oversees the workers who will take care of the patient.

5. Refers the senior to a geriatric specialist for a formal evaluation.

6. Arranges for appointments with different doctors, as well as necessary transportation to these appointments.

7. After assessing the elderly for his or her physical needs and financial situation, makes the arrangements to transfer the senior, to a nursing home or assisted living facility.

8. Will evaluate all options of care available to the patient, under his or her individual conditions.

9. May, if needed, take over the role of a guardian, if there is no family to step in.

The case managers are usually paid between $50 to $200 per hour. Initial assessment session may cost between $150 and $350 dollars per session. There is nothing that the case manager does that you or a family member cannot do. But if you can't commit to the time and extra work, the expense may be worth it to have a case manager step in to help.

Before employing such a manager, you should consider a few questions in relation to your specific situation. Among the questions you should ask the manager is:

What services are you offering?
What are your credentials?
How long are you doing case managing?
Are you member of any relevant organization?
Are you affiliated with the local hospitals or health organizations?
What information do you look for in the initial assessment session?
By which means, and how often do you keep in touch with the family of the patient?
How often will you visit the patient?
Will you report to the family as to the patient's situation?
Can you offer references?
What are your fees?

Will you provide a monthly report detailing expenses, treatments, follow ups, etc.?

In general you need to evaluate your particular situation to decide if in fact you need a case manager, and if you can afford one, for the long run. They do fulfill a role in making the transfer to a residential situation for the elderly or the infirm. They know their way around the system, and make it easier for the family, as well as for the patient. But the cost may be high.

Your state's Office of the Aged can help you find a case manager. See our site for contact information for the Office of the Aged in your state: www.goldenyearsgolden.com .

Giving Care-How to be prepared

Although currently 35 million people provide care to the elderly and the sick in America, it is not always clear if the quality of the care is what it should be. Care-giving mostly just happens, it is not planned, and often the need for care comes as a surprise. Caring for a parent or a spouse is not easy, and in most cases we are ill prepared for the task.

The smartest thing to do is to be prepared in advance, which means that we should do some homework and be educated as to what options are out there to help us provide the care for our loved ones when the need presents itself. Here are few things you should look at initially:

1. For the care giving to be successful, all people involved need to get along. If compromise is needed, so be it.

2. One person needs to coordinate the caregivers; all papers to be filled out, such as medical papers, insurance, Medicare, etc, should be filled out by the person that is best at it.

3. Have a plan as to how the care should be provided, by whom, and what the sources of payment will be. Have a plan for increase of care needs, as level of illness advances.

4. Make sure that the caregiver has a support system to help him or her to deal with his or her own personal needs.

5. Seek out organizations, books, professionals, that can be sources of help, support, and recognition for the care you need and provide.

6. Plan ahead for situations in which the care giver may need help, and the help should be there, whether it is a home health aide, a family member, relative, friend, or neighbor.

7. Offer opportunities for the caregiver to express themselves; maybe keep a log of issues that relate to the work they are doing. Take their needs seriously.

8. Include the caregiver in social situations, with the patient, when possible, or without them. This will make them feel recognized for their work and appreciated.

The caregivers are divided for the most part, into three categories:

1. The first category is made up of people who provide care as professionals, such as aides and nurses, who are paid for their services, either by the patient, their family, or by governmental agency, insurance, pensions, veteran benefits, or other sources.

2. The second category includes family members, relatives and friends of the patient. People in this category provide the care that is needed mostly free of charge, and with much love. Caregivers can be young or old, but from different demographic studies, it seems that the weight of care-giving falls mostly on people born between 1946 and 1964, the very boomers who themselves are coming into the senior age group.

As their parents slow down and start to show signs of decline, they cannot avoid seeing their own future before them - their own needs, when they reach their parents' age.

3. The third category are caregivers who are familiar with the patient and who step in when care is needed but it cannot be provided by family. It can be a neighbor or someone that a friend or relative knows. At times there is a fee for such services.

In the cases of the second and third categories, the caregivers usually do not have the medical knowledge to deal with the care of the patient. It is essential that the caregiver becomes familiar with the medical history, as well as with the treatment that the patient receives. The following is a fairly simple set of guidelines to help the caregiver establish a smooth and effective pattern of care.

What you need to know if you are to take care of an elderly, or sick person:

1. Be familiar with the medical condition of the person. Keeps a written log with medical instructions outlining your role in the care.

2. Speak to family members, doctors, therapists, anyone who is involved or provides services to the patient. Make sure that you not only know what the problems are that you have to deal as part of the care you will provide, but also that you are informed as to the things that can go wrong.

3. Make sure that your responsibilities are well defined and are clear to you. If the patient is fully alert, it is advisable to have the in-service or instructions given to you by his or her doctor or other service giver, in the presence of the patient. The patient thereby is aware of the fact that his caregiver is well informed.

4. One should familiarize oneself with the patient's routines and daily schedule. It is important that the patient's routines are not interrupted. The wonderful part of living at home is that the patient is able to maintain his or her past routines and habits, assuming such habits are not detrimental to their health.

5. Maintain a calendar of all appointments, scheduled with the coordination of family, and plan ahead for transportation.

6. Be aware of dietary restrictions - plan ahead for meals and shopping. Work with a list. If you have any questions as to what food or how much of it a patient is allowed, check with the patient's doctor or family.

7. Be respectful of the patient's schedule, routines that she or he enjoys, such as a show they like to watch. Do not plan meals or baths that will interfere with patients' routine.

8. Set up backup supplies. Keep an active list that reflects weekly needs in the patient's home. Make sure that you have food on hand for two to three days, if weather does not permit shopping. Make sure that there is enough medication, and make sure to refill a few days before needed.

9. Follow the emergency plan in this book.

10. Keep a log for routines, such as sleeping habits, eating habits, etc. If you notice changes, such as the patient is eating less, or is sleeping less, is irritable, depressed, less communicative, etc., make sure to inform the patient's doctor, and/or family.

11. Develop a backup plan with the family, for days you are unable to provide the home care. There must be a plan in place for coverage at short notice, if you get sick or have an emergency in your family.

12. Display a list of emergency numbers, such as doctors, pharmacy, family members, neighbors, ambulance; if any items that the patient uses are delivered, such as sugar level measuring sticks, have the number of the supplier displayed with other important numbers.

13. Make sure that the patient is aware of the emergency plan, and if possible, practice it. Make sure that you and the patient know what to do in case of fire, for example. Make sure the patient knows what to do if alone at home at time of an emergency.

14. Make sure that you do not expose the patient to any contagious diseases. At any sign of illness, notify the doctor and the family.

15. Protect patient's property and do not ask or interfere in his or her financial matters. Provide receipts for all purchases; keep a notebook with detailed accountability of all expenses. Keep in mind that you are shopping for them and their diet, not for yourself and your eating habits.

16. In an emergency, dial 911 first, and then call the doctor and the family.

For home care arrangements to work long term, one should be aware of the personalities that come into play. If a patient is a quiet and withdrawn person, it may not work if the care giver is a very bubbly person, walking around the house, singing, and talking nonstop. It is likely that the patient will tire soon, and demand a different worker.

If the caregiver is found through a good agency, they will ask questions about the personality of the patient, and will place a worker who is compatible with the patient's personality and needs.

If the family seeks a worker on their own, the personality of the worker should be evaluated, and the worker should have a clear understanding of the type of personality that the patient will present.

What you would like to prevent is numerous changes of care workers. It is very disconcerting to the patient, as well as to the family, to retrain and adjust to a new person. It will be much more effective if you take your time in interviewing a few people, checking their credentials and references, and picking the most suitable one for the patient.

But, that said, we do not always have the time to make those decisions. As I've said before, do the best within your situation.

It is recommended that the person who is hiring the worker set guidelines for the caregiver. You should make sure that there are no tempting items around the house. Although, you always need to check the references of the worker, which the agency will do automatically, you still need to be safe.

Make sure that all financial documents are stored under lock and key, and are not freely accessible. Make sure that there are no large quantities of money kept in the house, unless it is in a safe. The same applies to jewelry. If there are valuables in the patient's home, make sure the worker knows it, and is clearly accountable for it.

The one overseeing the worker, should visit the home of the patient regularly, and speak to the patient and worker often. Make sure that when visiting you have time to speak to the patient freely, without the presence of the worker. Take the patient for a walk, or send the caregiver out for a chore. This will give you and the patient time to speak freely about the worker and the care he or she is giving to the patient. Make sure to make it clear to the patient that he or she can voice their feelings freely, with no retribution.

Always take patient grievances seriously. And act upon them. It is important that the patient knows that you take their side, and that you seriously consider what they say. They have to trust you completely.

When you are clearing any complaint with the worker, initially do it with out the patient present.

First, the worker will be free to express themselves on the issue. Second, the patient may feel uncomfortable to dealing with whatever the complaint is and presenting it to the worker.

From my experience working all these years with the aged, most problems are easily solved when the worker is made aware of what is troubling the patient. All they have to do is say to the patient: "Sorry, I did not know that this bothers you, no problem. I will do it the way you prefer it."

The most important issue when establishing home care, is that all sides understand, that mutual respect is a given and cannot be compromised. Do not treat an elderly or a sick person as a child, just because they are unable to fully care for themselves. I always say, they may be physically impaired, but they are not necessary lacking mentally.

The worker needs to respect the patient and their home, and act accordingly. In return, the worker should also be recognized and respected, for his or her work, and the role they play in the care of the patient.

There is a difference, between providing care for a few hours a day, a few days per week, and care that is given 24 hours per day, seven days a week. Care provided a few hours per day, or a few days a week, is usually given by one person. That means that the patient just has to get used to one person. All instructions are given to one person and follow-up is easy. Did they do the work, or not? The tasks are the responsibility of one person, and they know they are accountable for them. The friendship ties are established much easier between the patient and a single caregiver.

If, however, the patient requires 24-hour care, seven days a week, the care has to be divided among two or more workers. No one person will be able to work 7 days, 24 hours a day, without compromising the patient's care and their own health.

In such a case, two caregivers are needed and some agencies will even staff a case with 3 workers, because that will avoid paying the workers overtime. (In the home health care business, if a worker works more than 40 hours a week, he or she is entitled to overtime). You can demand that the agency only staff two workers. Most of the time, the agency will comply with that demand.

Language and familiarity with the patient's cultural background is also very important. We do not want the patient to get upset because the caretaker did not, for instance, maintain the kosher practices in the kitchen. So it is important that all those special customs and practices are respected by the worker.

One of the most frequent problems that occur in patient's home care is food issues. It is perfect if your parent is Jewish, and you find a worker who is Jewish, or your parent is Italian, and you find a worker who is Italian and familiar with Italian cooking. But in most cases, you will not find a person to take care of your loved one who is the same nationality or religion.

So in most situations, there is a great deal of adjustment that has to be made on both sides. This is not only a problem that is present in home care. It is true for all situations where care is given, in nursing homes, residential facilities, as well as in assisted living. But it is more pronounced in the home care situation, because the care is given on a one-to-one basis.

But if all the wrinkles are ironed out, the home situation is the easiest transition from independent living, to being provided assistance, or full care for the patient. Changes occur at a more gradual tempo, allowing the person to adjust slowly, without sudden drama.

One other issue that seems to occur in the initial stages of adaptation in home care is the need for the patient to get used to the constant presence of a stranger in his or her house. A worker comes to your home, he or she is there to care for you, yet this stranger makes decisions regarding your health, and your needs, and shares YOUR home with you. That is a situation where there is a great deal of getting used to.

A smart caregiver will step slowly into the role. He or she will respect the fact that the person that they are about to care of has been an independent person, caring and making all their decisions for themselves, and it is very difficult to give this independence up to another person. It doesn't matter if the other person is your child, relative, or a stranger.

Wherever and whenever it is possible, let the patient, or the sick person, have his or her input into their own care. If the caregiver is not a member of the patient's family, time should be devoted for familiarization. After the elderly person accepts the caregiver, the care giving will be fully beneficial. Otherwise there will be negative tension that will affect the well-being of both the patient and the caregiver.

As mentioned previously, you need to have a legal document in place that will allow you to have the legal right to make medical decisions for your parent or loved one. Or you need to empower someone to make the medical decisions for you, when you are unable to do so yourself. That legal instrument is called "health care proxy". You will find a detailed description of this document in the chapter in this book dealing with the legal situations.

Assessing Workers in Residential Facilities and in Private Homes

Care Givers in Residential Facilities:

If an aide cares for your loved one in any of the previously mentioned residential situations, then you will not do the hiring and you will have no control as to who will take care of them. Visit the place you are screening, and talk to aides on the floor, rather than taking the routine tour with a guide designated by the facility.

Watch how the workers interact with the residents, preferably without them knowing that they are being watched. Just think, your parent might be there, among them. What you should look for is the tone in which the patients are being spoken to. Are the workers sensitive and caring when interacting with the residents? Are the aides physical, touching the patients roughly, and are they rushed, and in a hurry? If at times the aide does her job well, but is too strict and harsh, you do not want that for you parents.

As you will find with other residential options, here too you need to take time to examine the places well and objectively and ask yourself if your loved one will be happy there. He or she is likely to spend the rest of their life in that place.

If you are considering one of the residential options, ask if all staff members that are directly involved with the daily activities of the residents are licensed and certified for the tasks they perform. Are the workers screened for criminal background? Are they well trained? Does each worker receive an annual physical check-up?

Most places expect the potential resident, or his or her family member, to ask those questions. But if they are not forthcoming with their answers, leave, and look for another place.

Ask for the ratio of aides to patients. Check if the facility follows regulation of the given state you are in, and bathes the patients in a timely manner. Also question if, during staff members' vacations, the number of workers remains unchanged, and the care provided to the patient is not affected.

No matter how beautiful the facility, what is most important is the quality of care provided for the patients and if the residents are happy in the facility. Visit more than once and at different times of the day, as well as on weekdays and weekends, to see the servings and the feedings of different meals. See if there are enough personnel to serve and feed the residents.

The above suggestions are for workers in residential and nursing homes facilities. However, if you are looking for a home health aide to provide care for you, or your parent, the following suggestions will be of help to you.

Care Giver in your home

The first thing you want to look at is you parent's medical situation and if the care at home will meet your parent's needs. Is your parent ill? To what extent is your parent able to care for themselves, and how much does he or she need the help of the aide? Can your parent direct the home health aide, or does the direction need to come from you, or the agency that is providing the aide? Is your parent able to take his or her own medication or is there a need for reminder?

The next thing you need to look at is the cost of a home health aide. You need to know the cost in terms of long servicing; at the initial stage you may be able to cut costs, if your parent does not need full time care. There is a significant difference in cost if only eight hours per day of coverage is needed.

Then, if this option is suitable for you financially, you should do some research to find the most suitable aide for your parent. Where do you begin? There are different sources, which can help you to find the right aide. If you should be fortunate and receive a recommendation through a friend or a local doctor, it may be the easiest way, but most of us have to actively look for an aide. Some people put an ad in the paper, but then you have to interview, which is time-consuming and check the applicants' backgrounds and references. And you need to do a very thorough job. You will be leaving your loved one, as well as all that he or she owns and is dear to them, in the aide's care.

If you decide to go with an agency, however, you need to make sure it is an agency licensed by the health department in your state. If you or your parents have long-term home care insurance that will cover this service, you need to clear with the insurance company if the agency providing home care needs to be not only licensed, but also certified. Just to clarify that briefly, all home agencies have to be licensed, but not all need to be, or are certified.

In New York State for example, Medicare and Medicaid, as well as most insurance companies, require the agency to be certified, not only licensed.

If you are lucky enough to have long-term care insurance, check if the payments are made directly to the agency or if the insurance company will send the payments to you so that you have to pay the agency. As we all know, insurance companies do not pay very quickly, so you need to be sure to have enough money to cover the cost of the home care up front.

It is also possible that the insurance policy covers only part of the daily cost of the home care; you will have to supplement the rest. The best option is to have the insurance company pay the agency directly. And if needed, you pay the difference for which you are liable, to the agency.

If your worker comes to you through an agency, the agency should provide all the insurance that the state regulations require. But if you hire directly, you must fulfill all of the state' requirements. For your own protection, you will need workmen's compensation insurance, liability, and to make sure that your home insurance covers a home health aide present for home care. Check with your accountant if you need to deduct Social Security and Medicare directly or if your employee is personally responsible for the payment. But either way your responsibility is to make sure that if something happens to the home care worker, such as a physical injury or illness, you will not be held financially liable.

When hiring a home health aide, you should make sure that language is not a barrier in communication - if the patient and the caregiver do not understand one another the arrangement will never work. Aside from the aggravation that will be a constant outcome of miscommunication, it will also be a concern should there be an emergency. In my agency, I had aides that came for interviews, looking for employment, and aside from being trained in this country as home health aides, (at times courses were given in Polish and Russian), some had been nurses and doctors in their own country; yet I could not employ them due to the fact that they were unable to communicate in English. But in the cases where patients spoke Polish or Russian, those workers may have been perfect for them.

It is also advisable to in-service the worker periodically as to what their daily responsibilities are. If there is more than one worker, coordinate that the workload of chores and responsibilities so that it is equally shared.

It is true that the night worker is not going to take the patient to the park or go shopping, but the night aide can do laundry, iron, and maybe clean the bathroom. Sharing chores lowers the tension between workers. If tension between the workers develops, then without fail, it will affect the environment in which your loved one lives.

Some of the families of patients who receive home care like to give the aides gifts, out of gratitude for the care they provide to their loved ones. I personally always maintained that if the worker is paid fairly, there is no need to tip them and give gifts. But for holidays, if you choose to give a gift to the aide, it should be small, and all aides working on this case should receive gifts similar in value and size.

Gifts in general, monetary gifts in particular, build expectations on the worker's part. As the time they work for you, or your parent, is longer, they may expect larger and larger gifts. Thus, it is my recommendation that you do not give monetary gifts; make it a gift of an item of clothing, baskets of eatable goods, or some toiletries, such as perfume, etc.

Much more important is to express to the worker your appreciation for his or her work, to write a letter to the worker's agency to commend them of their good work so their supervisor is aware of their dedication to their client and their work. Most of us take the worker who takes care of us or our parent for granted, assuming this is their job, and they are paid for it. But in reality, we should recognize and acknowledge their work and commitment. Home care, good home care, is like nursing, i.e. it requires an emotional investment on the part of the worker.

In my experience during the many years that I worked with the elderly, I have seen a great deal of bonding between aides and patients, and their family members. It is natural human behavior that over time relationships become close and very personal, and such a relationship between the patient and his or her caregiver should not threaten the family.

I have seen the closeness that develops between the personal worker and the patient and the family, with the worker becoming an integral part of the family. Nonetheless, we should still maintain supervision. While we always should respect the worker, trust their ability to provide the proper care for our parent, it should be clear as to what the responsibilities should be, as well as the obligations on the aide's part.

The patient or family member involved with the care of the patient should be discouraged from keeping large amounts of money in the house. Valuables and important documents should be put in a safe place and not just out of fear of theft. When the patient becomes forgetful, he or she may misplace such items, and forget where they have put them, at times blaming the aide for taking them. This will cause tensions, until the misplaced item is found.

If the family is involved, they have to provide the worker with the information that the worker needs to give the patient the best possible care. The aide needs to know the medical status of the patient. If there are any nutritional restrictions, the worker should be informed of them and should follow them when preparing the meals for the patient.

The worker also needs to follow the doctor's instructions regarding physical restrictions and any other special care that their patient will need. The worker should feel the support of the family, and have open channels of communication with them; this will improve the quality of care the patient receives. If the patient does not have close relatives, the agency should oversee what the family would have.

Workers that work for a few years for the same person tend to burn out. At times it is enough to provide the worker with a few weeks of vacation, but in some cases it requires change - bringing in a new aide, who is energized and able to do all that is required of him or her.

To identify the burnout factor, watch if the caregiver exhibits moodiness or calls in sick often at a steadily increasing rate. If you see them being abrupt, short fused, and indifferent to the patient, those are tell- tale signs. If you notice some neglect, even as minor as your parent staying in bed longer or going out less and being less socially engaged, those also are signs.

As inconvenient as it may be to have a new aide introduced to your parent, and to adapt to all the routines that make up your parent's day, it is still a must, because having a burnt-out personal caregiver is more harmful to them. I would recommend, whenever it is possible, having two aides sharing a case, so if one worker has to be replaced, there is always one worker who the patient is familiar with. The change may be less dramatic.

Chapter 8 –
Financial-Know what you're doing

One of the biggest worries that the elderly have are the financial issues that they have to deal with daily. Very few of us have the luxury of retiring without any worries. The given formulas that have become standard for most exports on retirement state that one needs to base his or her future retirement on 75 to 85 percent of their current income.

Those are very general numbers that are basically based on maintaining a fairly similar level of living, with the curtailment of monthly expenses. For example, if you own a home, especially a large one, the upkeep and maintenance is very costly; thus downsizing your home may make a big difference in your monthly expenses.

For the many Americans who reach retirement age and are forced to live the rest of their lives on their Social Security entitlement, and possibly their monthly pensions check, the following chapter may be of very little interest. But for others, and I do hope a great deal of you, this chapter will provide an overview of the field of investment.

It is sort of a basic 101-level quick course on the subject. It is no substitute for the need to review all investments, with relation to your specific needs and abilities. And the best would be to seek out a good broker, or a financial planner, hopefully one that is highly recommended by someone you trust.

The following will help you to understand the general options that are available to you, and what the different investments consist of. My husband and I, with the advice of our financial advisor are taking advantage of many of the investment options mentioned here.

Personal finance – Investments made easy

There are thousands of stocks and dozens of ways to invest. In this chapter we will explain personal investments in a very simple way, to help you make educated and correct investment decisions in the future.

We all want our money to last forever, or at least as long as we need it. We want our money to grow every year, and make a decent percentage yield. And of course, we want it provide us with a steady income.

Now that we know what we want, it is very important to know what we do not want. It is desirable that we do all that is possible to shy away from losses and trouble.

1) We do not want to invest in a single stock that fluctuates sharply up or down every day. The potential of loss is high and it is not in our favor.

2) We want to stay away from high fees and high commissions; 2 percent or higher are too much.

3) If a broker or financial advisor promises 20 percent or more profit on an annual basis, please show him the door.

4) We do not want to time the market. Investments in the market should be for at least five consecutive years.

5) Do not put everything in one basket. Investments should be diversified in a few options.

6) Private company bonds offer high yields, but they can be too risky.

Now that we have an idea of what we should not do, let's start working on what we should do. We will start with few basic explanations about major investments channels. We will not include mutual funds because they have high fees in general, and they are too segmented. (The majority of them are heavily concentrated on one sector of the market.) They can drop in value a few consecutive years in a row. Our goal is to make money every single year.

Here are some recommended investments:

Fixed Income

Banks CDs (certificate of deposit)

Certificate of deposit is short- or medium-term, interest-bearing, FDIC-insured, debt instrument offered by banks and savings and loan institutions. CDs offer higher rates of return than most comparable investments do, in exchange for tying up invested money for the duration of the certificate's maturity. Money removed before maturity is subject to a penalty. CDs are low-risk, low-return investments, and are also known as "time deposits," because the account holder has agreed to keep the money in the account for a specified amount of time, anywhere from three months to six years.

Bonds

A bond is a piece of paper that shows a person has agreed to loan money to the U.S. government. The government uses the money to help pay its bills. Why do people buy bonds? Because it's easy! You can buy Series EE bonds and Series I Bonds from most banks or credit unions.

There are a few types of bonds, like the aforementioned corporate bonds, that are too risky. Here is a list of bonds guarantee by the US Government or local municipalities:

Bond Basics: Different Types of Bonds

Government bonds

In general, fixed-income securities are classified according to the length of time before maturity. These are the three main categories:

Bills: Debt securities maturing in less than one year.

Notes: Debt securities maturing in one to 10 years.

Bonds: Debt securities maturing in more than 10 years.

Marketable securities from the U.S. government, known collectively as Treasuries, follow this guideline and are issued as treasury bonds, treasury notes and treasury bills (T-bills). Technically speaking, T-bills aren't bonds because of their short maturity. All debt issued by Uncle Sam is regarded as extremely safe, as is the debt of any stable country.

The debt of many developing countries, however, does carry substantial risk. Like companies, countries can default on payments.

Treasury bonds are issued in terms of 30 years and pay interest every six months until they mature. When a treasury bond matures, you are paid its face value. The price and yield of a treasury bond are determined at auction. The price may be greater than, less than, or equal to the face value of the bond. Treasury bonds are sold in treasury direct (but not in legacy treasury direct), and by banks, brokers, and dealers.

Municipal bonds known as "munis", are the next progression in terms of risk. Cities don't go bankrupt often, but it can happen. The major advantage to munis is that the returns are free from federal tax. Furthermore, local governments will sometimes make their debt non-taxable for residents, thus making some municipal bonds completely tax-free. Because of these tax savings, the yield on a muni is usually lower than that of a taxable bond. Depending on your personal situation, a muni can be a great investment on an after-tax basis.

Annuities are a recommended investment, but first check fees and commissions, as well as how the broker/bank makes their money from your annuity. If there are excessive up-front fees - 4-5 percent - or commissions on the back end of the annuity after the maturity, be aware that it will lower your profits by at least 1-3 percent of the promised rate.

Please be extremely cautious when banks offer 2 to 3 percent over the fed interest rate for the first year. It is a hook. For rest of the duration of the annuity – an averaged of five or ten years - will be less than the promised rate, and after the bank fee or commissions are deducted, you will not find it as attractive as it first looked.

Here are some of the different types of annuities:

Fixed vs. Variable Annuities

In a fixed annuity, the insurance company guarantees the principal, and a minimum rate of interest. In other words, as long as the insurance company is financially sound, the money you have in a fixed annuity will grow and will not drop in value. The growth of the annuity's value and/or the benefits paid may be fixed at a dollar amount or by an interest rate, or it may grow by a specified formula. The growth of the annuity's value and/or the benefits paid does not depend directly or entirely on the performance of the investments the insurance company makes to support the annuity. Some fixed annuities credit a higher interest rate than the minimum, via a policy dividend that may be declared by the company's board of directors, if the company's actual investment, expense and mortality experience is more favorable than was expected. Fixed annuities are regulated by state insurance departments.

Money in a variable annuity is invested in a fund—like a mutual fund - but it is only open to investors in the insurance company's variable life insurance and variable annuities. The fund has a particular investment objective, and the value of your money in a variable annuity—and the amount of money to be paid out to you—is determined by the investment performance (net of expenses) of that fund. Most variable annuities are structured to offer investors many different fund alternatives. Variable annuities are regulated by state insurance departments and the federal Securities and Exchange Commission.

Types of Fixed Annuities

An equity-indexed annuity is a type of fixed annuity, but it looks like a hybrid. It credits a minimum rate of interest, just as a fixed annuity does, but its value is also based on the performance of a specified stock index—usually computed as a fraction of that index's total return.

A market-value adjusted annuity is one that combines two desirable features—the ability to select and fix the time period and interest rate over which your annuity will grow, and the flexibility to withdraw money from the annuity before the end of the time period selected. This withdrawal flexibility is achieved by adjusting the annuity's value, up or down, to reflect the change in the interest rate "market" (that is, the general level of interest rates) from the start of the selected time period to the time of withdrawal.

Other Types of Annuities

All of the following types of annuities are available in fixed or variable forms:

Deferred vs. Immediate Annuities

A deferred annuity receives premiums and investment changes for payout at a later time. The payout might be in a very long time; deferred annuities for retirement can remain in the deferred stage for decades.

An immediate annuity is designed to pay an income one time after the immediate annuity is bought. The time period depends on how often the income is to be paid. For example, if the income is monthly, the first payment comes one month after the immediate annuity is bought.

Fixed Period vs. Lifetime Annuities

A fixed period annuity pays an income for a specified period of time, such as ten years. The amount that is paid doesn't depend on the age (or continued life) of the person who buys the annuity; the payments depend instead on the amount paid into the annuity, the length of the payout period, and (if it's a fixed annuity) an interest rate that the insurance company believes it can support for the length of the pay-out period.

A lifetime annuity provides income for the remaining life of a person (called the "annuitant"). A variation of lifetime annuities continues to provide income until the second one of two annuitants dies. No other type of financial product can promise to do this. The amount that is paid depends on the age of the annuitant (or ages, if it's a two-life annuity), the amount paid into the annuity, and (if it's a fixed annuity) an interest rate that the insurance company believes it can support for the length of the expected pay-out period.

With a "pure" lifetime annuity, the payments stop when the annuitant dies, even if that's a very short time after they began. Many annuity buyers are uncomfortable with this possibility, so they add a guaranteed period, essentially a fixed period annuity, to their lifetime annuity. With this combination, if you die before the fixed period ends, your beneficiaries continue to collect the income until the end of that period.

Zero Coupon Bonds

Zero coupon bonds are bonds that do not pay interest during the life of the bonds. Instead, investors buy zero coupon bonds at a deep discount from their face value, which is the amount a bond will be worth when it "matures" or comes due. When a zero coupon bond matures, the investor will receive one lump sum equal to the initial investment plus interest that has accrued.

The maturity dates on zero coupon bonds are usually long-term and many don't mature for 10, 15, or more years. These long-term maturity dates allow an investor to plan for a long-range goal, such as paying for a child's college education. With the deep discount, an investor can put up a small amount of money that can grow over many years.

Investors can purchase different kinds of zero coupon bonds in the secondary markets that have been issued from a variety of sources, including the U.S. Treasury, corporations, and state and local government entities.

Because zero coupon bonds pay no interest until maturity, their prices fluctuate more than other types of bonds in the secondary market. In addition, although zero coupon bonds do not pay any interest until they mature, investors may still have to pay federal, state, and local income tax on the imputed or "phantom" interest that accrues each year. Some investors avoid paying the imputed tax by buying municipal zero coupon bonds (if they live in the state where the bond was issued), or purchasing a few corporate zero coupon bonds that have tax-exempt status.

The most recommended types are:

Zero Coupon Treasury Bonds

There are zero coupon bonds issued by the U.S. Treasury, corporations, and state and local government jurisdictions. Zero coupon Treasury bonds are generally considered the safest zero coupon bonds, backed by the full faith and credit of the U.S. government.

Municipal Zero Coupon Bond

These are issued by state and local governments and are usually exempt from federal and state taxes in their state of issue. They provide a convenient way to meet the goals of high tax bracket investors who get an after-tax benefit from the lower interest rates of tax-free municipals.

ETFs – Exchange-Traded Funds

Exchange-traded funds, or ETFs, are index funds that trade just like stocks on major stock exchanges. Want to invest in the market quickly and cheaply? ETFs are the most practical vehicle. They help the investor focus on what is most important, choice of asset classes.

All the major stock indexes have ETFs based on them, including:

- Dow Jones Industrial Average

- Standard & Poor's 500 Index

- NASDAQ Composite

Diversification

Because each ETF is comprised of a basket of securities, it inherently provides diversification across an entire index.

There are ETFs for large US companies, small ones, real estate investment trusts, international stocks, bonds, and even gold. Pick an asset class that is publicly available and there is a good bet that it is represented by an ETF, or will be soon.

ETFs differ fundamentally from traditional mutual funds, which do not trade midday. Traditional mutual funds take orders during Wall Street trading hours, but the transactions actually occur at the close of the market. The price they receive is the sum of the closing day prices of all the stocks contained in the fund. Not so for ETFs, which trade instantaneously all day long and allow an investor to lock in a price for the underlying stocks immediately. ETFs are economical to buy and especially to maintain over the long-run, making them especially attractive for the typical buy-and-hold investor.

Lower costs

Expenses can have a significant impact on returns for investors. ETFs, in general, have significantly lower annual expense ratios than other investment products. ETFs are less likely to experience high management fees, because they are index-based, not "actively" managed. And, since they trade on an exchange, ETFs are insulated from the costs of having to buy and sell securities to accommodate shareholder purchases and redemptions.

Although investors must pay a brokerage transaction to purchase them, with discount brokers this becomes negligible with sizable trades. There are a few easy-to-avoid pitfalls to watch out for. Tax effects are also not to be ignored, and ETFs perform well after taxes.

Tax efficiency

ETFs, like index funds in general, tend to offer greater tax benefits because they generate fewer capital gains due to low turnover of the securities that comprise the portfolio. Generally, an ETF only sells securities to reflect changes in its underlying index. Exchange trading of ETFs further enhances their tax efficiency. They can be margined; options based on them allow for various defensive (or speculative) investing strategies.

Dividend opportunities

Dividends paid by companies, and interest paid on bonds held in an ETF, are distributed to ETF holders, minus expenses, on a pro rata basis. Not all companies will pay dividends.

Their safety as a securities instrument (considered separately from the safety of any particular asset class they might represent) is considered the same as stock certificates themselves. Internally, ETFs are far more complex entities than mutual funds. A fascinating combination of players, including brokers, money managers, and market specialists combine to make them run smoothly. Legally, ETFs are a class of mutual fund as they fall under many of the same Securities Exchange Commission rules that traditional mutual funds do. But their different structure means that the SEC has imposed requirements that are different from traditional mutual funds in how they are bought and sold.

ETFs are index funds at heart, so investors are encouraged to study the philosophy of index investing - which downplays individual stock picking in favor of buying a sort of snapshot of specific financial market. But unlike most traditional index funds, investors need not take a passive, buy-and-hold approach. ETFs are also becoming favorites of hedge funds and day traders who like to pull the trigger frequently. Both types of investors may coexist and, in fact, strengthen each other by lowering overall transaction costs.

Now you may be ready to make sense of it all. Please note that all these investments come with no fees or commissions, or very minimal commission that caps at 0.75% a year. This method enables the investor to make as much money as possible, without losing unnecessary percentages due to high fees and commissions.

The key to receive interest/income every single year is based on both the type of investments described above and diversification. It is a good idea for one to invest 40-50 percent of their portfolio in fixed income and the rest in equities.

On the fixed income portion, one should have a mix that includes banks CDs, bonds, annuities (proceed with caution, ask all the questions), Zero coupons bonds, or other investments. The fixed income segment will increase in value about 5 percent a year guaranteed.

On the **equities** portion one should invest in the broad market ETFs index funds. Buy a few of the ETFs to cover most of the market. There are hundreds of ETFs. Shy away from ETFs that concentrate on single segments of the market such as energy, oil and gas, metals, and real estate, etc. Here are a few sample ETFs that cover broad segments of the market:

iShares: Spider S&P 500 (Amex SPY) – imitates S&P 500, which include the biggest companies also known as "blue chips."

Dow Diamonds ETF (Amex: DIA): The investment objective of the fund is to provide investment results that generally correspond to the price and yield performance of the Dow Jones Industrial Average. This offers a good dividend yield of 3.36 percent.

iShares: RUSSELL 2000 Idx (NYSE ARCA:IWM)-Index fund that measures the performance of the small-capitalization sector of the U.S. equity market.

Midcap SPDR trust; 1 (Amex MDY): 400 mid-cap companies. Imitates the S&P 400.

iShares: S&P SC 600 Idx (NYSE ARCA:IJR): 600 small-cap companies. The fund seeks investment results that correspond generally to the price and yield performance.

Powershares: QQQ Trust (NASDAQ GM:QQQQ): The investment objective of the trust is to provide investment results that generally correspond to the price and yield performance of the component securities of the NASDAQ-100 Index.

The equities above will generate between 5 and 15 percent a year on average during the course of five to 10 years). The combination between the fixed income (5 percent) and the equities (5 to 15 percent) will generate about 7 to10 percent every year.

It is recommended at the age of 60 to reduce equity holdings by 10 percent every five years and shift it to the fix income portion of your investment.

Warning: Please do not check the market every day. It is in constant flux, and sometimes drops considerable for a short period of time. You will be discouraged and upset if you take a daily approach.

We recommend checking your statement once a month and checking the results by quarters, not daily or a monthly. You are in it for the long haul. The method represented will give you peace of mind; after the first purchases, sit and relax; your next move will be months from now. Let the money work for you. With some patience, you'll see great results.

To maximize profits one should evaluate the equity portion of the portfolio once a year. Consult with a broker and/or financial advisor to check if there is a need to shift money from one ETF to another.

There are certain years that the large caps (blue chips) such as S&P 500 do better and some years the small ETFs perform better.

When investing for your retirement while you are still working, you can be a little bolder. But when investing after you actually retire, it is wise to be more conservative.

I hope that the above information is of benefit to you, and may help you to make the right decisions when investing for your retirement years, or at least help you to understand what your broker is telling you.

I think it will be wise to repeat that you should be careful. The baby boomers and their parents make a good target for all kinds of schemes, such as annuities that are unsuitable for the seniors, as well as ones with over-hyped investment returns. Be careful and suspicious of any sales pitch that promises unrealistic returns, such as 12 percent or higher.

Before signing up with a broker, check their background, for which you can use the Finra's Broker Check tool (www.finra.org) . If there any disciplinary actions taken against the broker or if she or he has been moving from one financial institution to another frequently, it should raise a red flag.

Open an account with a reputable and independent financial institution, and never write your investment check to an individual – always write it to the financial institution.

All investment decisions should be made without pressure. When I meet a broker for investment, I never have my checks with me. I go home, think it over, and talk it over with my kids, my husband and my financial adviser. If the broker pressures me to make the decision right there, because the deal will not be there the next day, I walk away from the "deal" as well as the broker.

Chapter 9 –
Legal Issues – Self Protection

General Legal Issues and Elder Fraud

Besides insurance coverage, safety, and health care provisions, there are many other potential dangers that the elderly and their loved ones need to worry about. As our society becomes more technologically dependent and criminals become more sophisticated in their techniques, it becomes very essential that we stay one step ahead and establish proper protection for seniors.

According to congressional estimates, telemarketing fraud cheats American citizens out of about $40 billion annually. The American Association of Retired Persons says that half of those victims are above the age of 65.

Although the general population is vulnerable, the elderly are often, unfortunately, easy marks for scammers. It is hard to come up with the exact numbers of elderly victims, because there are so many different types of fraud perpetrated against them, and many seniors do not report the crime, often because they are unaware that they were victims of fraud. Another reason for not having accurate numbers of fraud victims is the fact that the legal definition of what constitutes fraud is not exact.

To define fraud, we can say that a good or service is promised and it is not delivered. If there is a signed agreement or contract and it is not fulfilled, then it is easy to prove that fraud was perpetrated. It is difficult to prove fraud, however, when the agreement is verbal or when written agreement is very vague or full of loopholes.

Our seniors grew up in a different era. There were fewer opportunities to trick them, and today, with so much automation, it is fairly easy to take advantage of a trusting person and retrieve information that can be used to gain access to his or her money.

As a child or a guardian of an elderly person, you have to advise them that no personal information, such as address, date of birth, Social Security number, or any banking and credit card information should be given over the phone. And anyone requesting such information over the phone should be politely cut off. No purchases should be made on the phone and credit card information should only be given out when the senior him or herself initiated the call. Some of the calls can sound very sophisticated, and at times the caller will claim that the call is from their bank or from a government office, and they only want to update the person's personal information. It is important, however, that no personal information is given. Government agencies do not update their data through telephone calls. Some scammers will pretend they are from such offices, just to gain personal and financial data to use in effort to gain access to a victim's money. If someone calls to requesting personal or financial information, the proper response is, "thank you, good bye," before hanging up the phone.

When I was running a home care agency, I encountered some very sophisticated scams, many outright illegal and some so well disguised, it was hard for even a trained professional to realize they were scams.

Another popular scam targeting the elderly, especially those living alone, is the mailing of fake invoices that look like bills, particularly medical bills. It is hard for seniors to remember which doctors they had visited, or know which laboratories were used for their blood tests. If the bill is vague as to the services provided, lists code numbers of tests rather than verbal descriptions, and the dates of services is several months past, I can assure you that younger people would not remember if they actually had a given test, either.

It is important to keep some kind of record of appointments with doctors and tests that were taken, so you are able to verify bills that you or your loved one receives. If anything looks out of the ordinary, or if the name of the medical office does not look familiar, or the payment envelope lists a post office address, double check everything. That's usually is a giveaway.

With access to a computer, it doesn't take a master criminal to print an official-looking document that looks as if it came from a printing shop. And as the crooks are becoming more and more innovative, they have started mailing counterfeit utility bills – invoices that look exactly like gas, electric, and telephone bills. You need to be alert to the fact that scams are out there, and the scammers are getting better.

While many neighbors are good and caring people, there may be few among them that are con artists masquerading as helpful souls who volunteer to help a senior, until they gain the person's trust. Then, they slowly take advantage of their elderly victim. Do not give neighbors or friends power of attorney, unless you are very sure about their intentions. Any attorney will tell you that, ideally, you should have two people looking after your affairs. This way each one will be accountable to the other.

Many elderly people develop friendly and warm relationships with the home health aides who work for them, especially if the aide has been working for them a long time. Nonetheless, one should maintain a business relationship with the worker, and not involve them in financial issues. A home health aide should be your health aide and not your financial adviser. A good agency will in-service their workers, to keep them from getting involved in money matters of their clients.

Another favorite with the scammers are donations. We've all receive envelopes that on the outside look like standard fundraising organization envelops. It they have certain words in the organization's name, such as cancer, lung diseases, heart disease, etc., it may look authentic enough to seem like a real charitable organization. In general, people are trusting, and believe that any organization going to the trouble of sending an appeal is legit, and the funds do go to the causes that they advertise. But be prudent and check with the Attorney General's office in your state to find out if the fund is legitimate.

There are countless charitable organizations that do good work, and they subsist on donations and bequests. I am not suggesting that seniors should not support any number of reputable organizations and foundations, but a donor should screen them well. It is not a good idea to allow an organization to be an executor, or grant the organization a power of attorney. The organizations that stand to gain after your death tend to have an agenda of their own that does not usually reflect yours.

If an organization is an executor over your estate, it should not also be a health proxy designated to make decisions on your health issues. The person you designate to make the health decisions, the one who will make life and death decisions should not have a financial stake in your life or death. And as I state in the chapter dealing with specific legal issues, you should leave specific direction to the person designated to carry out your living will and health proxy..

In 2006, according to adult protective services statistics, over half a million cases of abuse of the elderly were reported. That included neglect and cruelty of all sorts, physical and mental abuse, larceny, and telemarketing theft; 89 percent of the abuse happened in the person's own home. Some of the abusers may well be the ones caring for the victims, or a family member. As I said before, many of the elderly who are abused are afraid to report those abuses.

Meanwhile, the federal government remains ineffective. There are some bills that may be introduced to the Senate that will provide millions of dollars for research and programs to protect the elderly. If passed, the money will be used to strengthen the existing protective services, and to better educate the staff of such agencies to provide services greatly needed by the elderly at the professional level.

Provisions in these bills will provide tools for the police and prosecutors necessary to deal with criminals preying on the elderly with much heavier criminal punishments than is currently the norm.

Telemarketing fraud once was limited to small-scale crooks, but now it has become a global enterprise preying on the general public. In recent years these rings have targeted the elderly, the very population that is the most vulnerable. With every government agency, every financial institution, every store, and every school compiling computerized data, every transaction or registration exists in a database. And all this data can be kept forever.

Companies like InfoUSA, one of the largest compilers of consumer data, have carved a market selling lists of this data to basically whoever will pay for them. In May 2007, **The New York Times** reported the sale of lists of "Elderly Opportunity Seekers" being advertised. This was a list of 3.3 million seniors, offered to buyers looking for ways to make money. "The suffering seniors" list, also for sale, offered 4.7 million names of seniors with cancer or Alzheimer's disease.

In that advertisement, the sellers promoted the vulnerability of seniors and pointed out to potential buyers how gullible the elderly can be. In other words, the elderly are a perfect target. And InfoUSA is not alone, there are many more legal companies like it, and more are being established every day.

Direct marketing has similarly bulldozed its way into our lives, with calls made at all hours of the day, disrupting dinners, holidays, and our favorite TV shows. Older Americans are perfect target for the aggressive, well-trained telemarketer; they are almost always at home and they are in no hurry to terminate the call - too well mannered to just cut the caller off and hang up the phone. To some seniors, a marketing call may be the only social call of the day. When you're lonely, a friendly voice on the other end of the line is very appealing – they may not realize that the caller wants something from them.

The number of scams against the elderly are on the rise; the Federal Trade Commission estimated that 11 percent of all telemarketing scams are carried out against people 55 years and older.

One popular scam used by telemarketers – whether legal or illegal – is to gain personal information by offering sweepstakes entries, tempting the seniors with hope of winning. A large number of the sweepstakes are fakes, only a ruse to gain the information about the person, as to his or her shopping habits, religion, and other personal data.

Criminals also focus on the elderly because they know that most the elderly victims will not be quick to complain, being embarrassed to tell their children the truth out of fear that they will put them in a nursing home. At times the elderly may even be forgetful, or may have initial stages of Alzheimer's, and do not even realized that their money has been stolen.

The government should force the banks to employ some safeguards to protect the elderly, and if large sums of money are withdrawn through electronic transfer or an unsigned check system, automatic notification should be sent to the senior's children, guardian, or attorney. Or in some cases, protective services should step in.

So if a telemarketer is very sympathetic, projects care and interest in the elderly on the other end of the phone, listening to stories about his or her life, kids, and problems, it does not take long before a trust bond is established between them, and the senior is ready to give all the information he is asked to reveal. The elderly person sees the caller not as a stranger, but as a friend, someone who genuinely cares.

Case # 14

Ms. R. was 89 years old when she called our agency for home care. She had gone through some minor surgery, and needed someone to be with her for a few days until she fully recovered. She had a wonderful demeanor and a life full of social activities. Like many of our patients, she lived independently, and without the support of a family. She had a few cousins, a niece, and a nephew. They were not especially close to her, and the contact with them was minimal.

When our aide started working with Ms. R., she was very vocal about not trusting her family and thinking that their only interest in her was the money she would be leaving them.

We noticed that a non-for-profit organization, visited Ms. R. regularly, bringing small gifts, and slowly gaining her trust. As was our policy, we did not interfere in the client's affairs, unless there is something illegal endangering to the client.

Ms. R. decided to maintain home care service, even though she bounced back from her surgery. Months went by and the service went smoothly, with Ms R. resuming her social life, going to senior centers, small trips, concerts, and religious services. The aide was always by her side.

One morning I received a phone call from a representative of the organization that was regularly visiting Ms. R. One of their administrators, in a very friendly voice, introduced herself and said that they have a very good relationship with Ms. R., and they are working toward having her appoint them as her guardians. This would transfer the management of her finances to them.

She proceeded to ask me how much our agency was charging Ms. R. for the services we provide. I refused to give her this information, stating that this was private information. "Don't worry; we will pay you twice as much, when we take over. And everyone will be happy."

I refused to continue the conversation, and hung up. I did inform Ms. R. about this call and advised her to let her lawyer know about this.

Some months went by, until one morning I received a call from Ms. R.; she was crying and told me, "Please come, they are forcing me to sign some papers." I caught a taxi, and ran up to her apartment, which was not very far.

In the apartment, a woman and a lawyer representing the organization were trying to explain to me that Ms. R. had asked them to take over the management of her financial affairs. All the while, Ms. R. kept repeating that she never said any such thing, and she may be old, but she is not crazy.

I asked Ms. R. "Do you want them to leave?" she said "yes." I proceeded to ask them to leave, and informed them that I will inform my client's attorney regarding what had just happened. I did just that, and as far as I recall, her attorney wrote a letter to the organization, stating that it is illegal and unethical to try to force an elderly person to sign legal papers without the presence of her attorney.

For a long time I kept thinking, what if I had not been there? What if she had no one to call? Most elderly people can be talked into or intimidated into doing things that may hurt them in the long run. And this was a so-called legitimate organization that was out to get control over her finances, and in turn, control over her life.

Federal, state and city governments need to establish a campaign that is simple and understandable for seniors, that teaches them how to protect themselves from such criminals. Many venues should be used to reach the elderly and convey this information, and that information should be repetitive, so the warning signs will be fresh in seniors' mind.

There can be a mailing campaign with literature warning the elderly. The government can send that information with their Social Security checks, explaining to seniors what should they do or not do when approached by suspicious persons. Another method could be printing a number to call to report any cases of financial fraud on the backs of milk cartons, just as currently is done for missing children. Medicare can send flyers with warnings to seniors in all their mailings. Warning posters can be posted in senior centers and retirement communities.

Here are some ways you or your parent can protect yourselves:

1. Say NO. You do not have to be liked by everyone, especially salespeople. It is okay to say no.

2. If it seems too good, it is. Nothing is given away for nothing If someone is trying to sell you a bill of goods, stop them from continuing: they'll sound more convincing the more time you give them to talk.

3. Telemarketers should be avoided at all cost. They are trained to confuse you, misinform you, and trick you into giving them your personal information. Over the phone, you can never know if it is a legitimate telemarketer representing a legitimate company, or a well- rained criminal. Just hang up the phone. A common trick a criminal uses is to tell the person on the phone that they are calling from their bank to clarify something about their account. Never give out account numbers, take the name and the phone number of the caller, say good bye and hang-up. Then go to your branch to check if there is a problem with your account.

4. Protect your personal information; never give any information if someone calls you. Even if you initiate the call, limit the amount of information you are giving out. It is especially important not to give out your Social Security number.

5. Never give your credit card information over the phone, except if you're the one initiating the call that involves paying a bill or making a purchase with a company you know and trust.

6. Be very careful buying from companies you are not familiar with, your purchased item may never arrive and your credit card information may be illegally used and sold to others.

7. Never use your credit card as a verification of your identity: crooks try hard to get your credit card information, even if you are not purchasing anything.

8. Do not let anyone pressure you to make a decision on the spot. Do not believe that the deal is only good for "now". Take your

time to think it over. Even if you intend to make the purchase, always leave yourself a day or two to think the deal over.

9. It is your right to ask as many questions as you need to. You should not be intimidated by anyone. If they are dismissive, not answering your questions or refusing to divulge information, hang up the phone. Believe me; you do not want to deal with this person.

10. Before you commit yourself to anything or sign anything, ask to see everything in writing. Read and reread everything before signing.

11. Seek out advice of a professional, a friend, or someone you know and trust before you commit your money.

12. Discard all mailings informing you of "prizes" you have won. They are just trying to trick you to purchase something you do not need. As the old saying goes, there's no such thing as a free lunch.

13. Never open the door for a door-to-door salesman. Some maybe legitimate sales persons, but many crooks will pretend to be salespeople to gain entry to your home. If someone knocks on your door telling you their car broke down and they need to make a phone call, or they need a glass of water because they do not feel well, do not open the door, especially if you are alone. Tell the person behind the door that you will call the local police to get them help and then do so. It is unfortunate that we should need to be so untrusting, but it's better to be safe than sorry.

14. Trust your instincts. When you have a bad feeling about something, it's usually right.

I will end this chapter with a case of fraud that one of our agency's patients had the misfortunate luck to experience.

Case # 15

Mrs. C. was 85 years old when our agency was hired by her son to provide home care for her. Up until that point, Mrs. C. lived on her own while her son lived in another state and traveled a great deal for his work.

He was relieved to have us step in and initially provide his mother with eight hours of care, seven days per week. She was very demanding and difficult to please, which took some time for the aides working with her to get used to. She called the agency day and night, and we seemed to provide direct or indirect care 24 hours a day.

Mrs. C. was suspicious and did not trust anyone, either in person or over the phone, which is why it was so unusual for her to be a victim of fraud. Nonetheless she became one.

A routine was established and she seemed to begin to trust the two aides who were caring for her. The number of hours that we provided home care increased, first to 12 hours per day, then to 24 hours. Basically, Mrs. C. was never left alone anymore. Our aides were well trained to ferret out fraudulent phone calls and attempts to swindle money from patients.

At some point, Mrs. C. was hospitalized with an irregular heart beat. The hospital allowed us to provide her regular aide only during the day. Therefore, she was on her own in the hospital room at night.

Within five days we brought the patient back home. A month later her son called me and asked if any of the aides working with his mother live in Florida. I did not understand what he meant, but told him that both aides lived in New York City.

He explained that he was billed by a credit company, from which he never had a credit card, for $18,000, for furniture and other household goods that were purchased in Florida. The credit card had been created in his mother's name.

His mother never had a credit card in her life, and throughout her life she never handled the family's finances - her husband had taken care of all the bills and check writing. After he passed away, her son took over the handling of all his mother's financial affairs.

I knew that my aides had nothing to do with the fraud, and they informed us that there were no suspicious calls in which Mrs. C. gave out any information on the phone to anybody that could have been used for opening a credit card account.

With the investigation that the credit card company pursued, it seemed that the personal information had been gotten from the hospital, while Mrs. C. was hospitalized. Who had penetrated the hospital records, and whether it was done by computer or through paper records, is not quite clear. She may also have been approached by somebody at the hospital and, thinking that the person was part of the hospital staff, may have given out some information. Either way, it seems that her Social Security number, name, address, and date of birth were accurately lifted.

In Mrs. C.'s case, all her incoming mail was forwarded to her son and he immediately acted upon this fraud. But often the target of fraud is a senior who has no one to verify the bills for correct charges, and many times will pay for things he or she never bought. Some of the seniors may also not know that they are not liable for purchases they have not made and, if contested, the credit card company will remove the charges from their account. It takes some calling and following up, but there is no need to rush and pay for it.

In many cases, no matter how careful we are, we still can be victims of fraud, but we can reduce the chance of it happening by being suspicious and cautious.

Legal Issues-Estate Planning

Talking about finances with our parents may be difficult, but avoiding the conversation may cause more problems, especially if their health is beginning to be an issue. Estate planning was once very simple. You had a will in place, and that was all you needed. Today it is more complicated, we are living longer, and our finances are invested in a variety of ways, thus we need to have much more complex estate planning set up.

And because we live longer and illnesses that were once a sure death sentence are now treatable, or acquired the status of chronic disease, we now need to build our estate planning with an emphasis on the long-term care costs. It has to be clear that the type of long-term care coverage should be evaluated according to your finances and needs.

Estate planning is highly misunderstood. It is perceived as something that only the wealthy need to focus on. But in actuality, everybody needs to plan for the future. Planning ahead is not only financially prudent, but it also helps you to develop a "blue print" to follow for future needs. Through such planning, you may be surprised to realize what you actual needs may be for your senior years, and this estate planning will make you aware if you are financially over or under your specific marker of needs.

Most people find it difficult to deal with financial issues that relate to their death. It is easy to procrastinate or ignore it entirely. It is a misconception that if we share legal ownership of all our possessions with our heirs, that ownership will automatically be transferred to them. This may be an expensive misconception. Although most people think of their distribution of assets after their death; one should also look at the possibility of distribution before death. One should consider that as a way of preserving the assets. It is wise to take advice from an estate planner and/or a good accountant.

It is important to understand that if one does not have a will, by law, the state has the right to step in and divide your property, with no consideration, or minimal consideration to the deceased's family. The state can select the heirs your money goes to, allow large sums to the tax collectors, and than charge your estate for this service. And those fees can be quite high. Yet even today, seven out of ten people have not had a will made up. The main reasons people do not have a will is their discomfort in dealing with the concept of their own death, or an indecisiveness as to how to divide their wealth. Most people in need of a will also worry about the cost of lawyers to prepare the will, yet the average cost of a will is between $300 and $500. A will should be reviewed every three to five years to make sure that it is updated to reflect your wishes and financial status. The lawyer should keep the original, while you should keep a copy.

Many people are relying more and more on the abundance of Internet sources that can provide them with a tool such as a will or a trust builder. For as little as $70 you can develop a will quite easily on a site called LegalZoom.com.

Recently, the numbers of legal sites have increased, and they are extremely sophisticated. They include not only do-it-yourself wills, but help with estate planning, as well. Estate planning can be costly and depends on how complicated the estate is. Living trusts can cost even higher. So if you are reluctant to pay an estate planner, you may consider the Internet option.

You have to follow the do-it-yourself, online instructions very carefully when you write a will or an estate planner. The signing of a will requires two signatures of witnesses, but it does not require those signatures to be notarized. As opposed to the will, the estate planning, trusts, and living trust almost always require witnesses and notarizing the documents to make them legally valid. Some of the regulations may vary from state to state, so make sure you check the requirements in the state in which you file the documents.

None of the self-filled documents need to be filed in court to make it legal, but it would be advisable to give a copy to your executors and your lawyer, if you have one, and let your family know where you are keeping the original.

As to the cost, Quicken WillMaker Plus has added living trusts to their site, as well as power of attorney, starting at a cost of $49.99 (www. nolo.com). Other sites that may concentrate on specific types of trusts such as Living Trusts on the Web, www.livingtrustontheweb.com, which charges about $149 for an individual, and $199 for a couple. Those prices were accurate at the time this book went to print.

Many experts advise that do-it-yourself estate planning is most suitable for people whose estate is worth less than $2 million, according to an Oct. 14, 2007 article in *The New York Times*. Above $2 million, the federal tax kicks in.

Estate planning not only provides for distribution after death, but may also provide protection for your money before you die. If you do not plan and leave written instruction as to what you want to be done for you if you become incapacitated, the state can come in and make the decisions for you. If your parent is hesitant and uncomfortable planning ahead, you may encourage him or her to do it in increments. Consult an estate planner who specializes in elder planning or someone they trust. It is important that they understand that their hard-earned money is protected for as long as they live, or as long as they are able to decide for themselves.

It is very important that the legal documents in which you leave your dear one's wishes are kept up to date. The will, for instance, will not negate other documents that may be in place, such as bank accounts that are set up in trust for someone and are not included in the will. Insurance policies that have a designated beneficiary will not be included in the will.

If a named beneficiary has died, and that beneficiary was not taken off the insurance policy, account, or trust, the court will intervene, and make the decisions, as to who gets what. This is the main reason why it is of utmost importance that you update your will or trusts regularly. The court may appoint an attorney to represent your interests; the attorney's fee will be charged to your estate.

It may be a good idea to set up a secondary beneficiary, especially if the first one is elderly. It will be beneficial to set up the will as clear as possible, to avoid any misunderstanding or conflict. This has to be done if you want the will to be carried out to your specifications. Review the will annually to make sure that all beneficiaries are still the ones to whom you want to leave your money.

You also need to verify that the executors you picked to carry out your wishes are still willing and able to fill this role. If the situation changes and that person is unable or unwilling to fill this role, you need to choose someone else.

If you choose to use an attorney to draw up a will, the cost can be as low as $250, for a simple will, to $750 and up, and the more complicated the will, the higher the cost. As for trusts and living wills, the cost can be $2,000 and up. Here too, shop around, and compare.

Note that the will becomes effective only after one's death. So if one is unconscious or mentally unable to make decisions, it does not mean the will is going to be probated. So for such scenarios you should establish other instruments to take care of your needs and protect your estate.

When writing a will or planning trusts, do not assume that all your heirs, family members, friends, and others whom you may want to leave part or all of your estate will get along and agree upon everything related to the probate of your estate. If you go on the assumption that people are not perfect and conflict is likely to take place, you should do all that it is in your power to minimize tensions among the people that will benefit from your estate. The best way to do that is to be as clear and specific as you possibly can. Providing copies of your will to everyone involved, is also helpful, thus they will know what to expect.

Estate Planning is easier to grasp when we understand the function of this tool and its terminology.

The Will

The will is an instrument to leave instructions on how an individual wants his or her estate to be distributed after their death. It may be set up to include a trust, and usually includes an executor.

From my experience with wills, it may be wise to have two executors for a will; it is for checks and balances. One executor can make decisions that may not fully reflect your wishes, or may stretch the power that you have put in his or her hands. If there are two executors, they are accountable to each other. The more explicit you are in the will, the fewer errors are made, and the easier it is to follow your wishes.

A will can be written on a notebook page, and as long as it is signed by two witnesses, it will be a legal instrument. Nonetheless, my advice to you will be to use a lawyer, and follow the formal legal pattern to avoid any loopholes that could leave an opening for legal procedures that could potentially disqualify your will and your wishes.

Trusts

Trusts come in many shapes, sizes, and forms; they can be structured to meet your special needs. But in general, all trusts have three elements: a grantor, a beneficiary, and a trustee. The following are short descriptions of the three:

The Grantor: The person or institution who transfers assets into the trust. If you are transferring assets into the trust for your children, for example, you are the Grantor.

The Beneficiary: The person or institution who will receive money or other assets from the trust, according to the terms you areestablishing in the trust.

The Trustee: A person or an institution that you designate to carry out the duty to manage, invest, and distribute assets in the trust. In all living trusts, all three elements are needed, but they need not be three different people. For example, a grantor may create a trust for tax or other reasons, in which he or she, can also be a trustee, and/or a beneficiary.

The directive instruments below are some of the ones you can use to serve your needs, and situation:

A Testamentary Trust

This is a trust that does not take effect until after the death of the creator of the will. This trust can be used if you choose not to leave the moneys to your heirs outright. When forming this trust, you may want to designate a trustee to manage the trust, and oversee the payout from trust, in the way you desire.

This type of trust may be good for someone leaving money to organizations or institutions. It also may be used for funds to be paid out over time, while the trust is invested and earning money.

An Irrevocable Trust

This is a trust which, once it is created, may not be revoked or amended by the person that establishes this trust. Most such trusts are used for income, gifts, or estate tax planning, are irrevocable in order to gain the tax advantages.

A Revocable Trust

This type of trust can be subject to being revoked or amended by the person who is establishing this trust. This type of trust is often used in cases when the primary objective is to maintain privacy during the grantor's life or after his or her death.

A Living Trust:

A living trust transfers property, stocks, and other possessions from one person to another. That is, to a living person. Using this instrument, one avoids probate and also is protected in case they are incapacitated. A revocable living trust gives the person creating the trust the right to change the terms of the trust, in part or the whole, or to dissolve the trust altogether. This type of trust is favored by many seniors, because it is not final by nature. The fact that the person devising it can change his or her mind makes it more appealing. As opposed to a will, this instrument isn't geared towards death specifically - rather it is designed to protect the living person.

A Charitable Remainder Trust

This type of trust is created as an irrevocable trust to provide income or annuity payments for a beneficiary. Often, the beneficiary is the grantor himself. When the trust expires, the remaining assets are transferred to a charitable organization, usually determined beforehand by the grantor.

Insurance Trust

This type of irrevocable trust holds life insurance policies on one or more individuals. It is often used to exclude life insurance proceeds from estate taxes. When the person who is insured dies, the trust receives, manages, and/or distributes the proceeds.

A Trustee and an Executor

A trustee and an executor can be a family member, friend, lawyer, or any trustworthy person who is charged with overseeing the execution of your will. The executor will distribute the will as per your written instructions, as well as pay any debts, taxes and expenses. The executer's responsibilities are concluded after the will is fulfilled and all possessions are delivered to whomever the author of the will designated.

The trustee manages the trust. The trustee continues to manage the trust for however long the trust is designated to exist.

A Letter of Instruction

This document, prepared for the beneficiaries of the will or trust, is meant to serve as a guide for closing out the affairs of the individual upon their death. This document should be consistent with the will or trust. It also should include direction and instructions as to the funeral and the list of people that the individual would like to be notified upon their death. It is also prudent to have a list of all the individual's possessions attached to that document.

A Durable Power of Attorney

This instrument gives another person the right to sign his name to any business transaction in your name; it also gives them the power over all your assets. This document can only be valid if it is prepared while the person signing over this power of attorney is fully competent mentally, and can be terminated at any time by written request.

Case # 16

Mr. V. was a sweet elderly person - already 96 years old when I met him. Alert and social, he loved his music and had a girlfriend with whom he went to concerts and shows. He lived independently, in a small apartment in a luxurious building in Manhattan. He still took long, slow walks around his neighborhood. Unfortunately, a slip on a wet patch on the sidewalk put an end to all of that.

After a lengthy stay in the hospital followed by time in a rehab center, the hospital's social worker had recommended my agency for his home care needs.

Mr. V. was a well-to-do person; he married late in life and had no children of his own and neither did his late wife. She, however, had a nephew and a niece. After his fall, Mr. V. life and daily routine changed. He required help with daily activities, such as bathing and dressing. His shopping and cooking had to be done by our aide. Since he had given over the control over his finances to his late wife's nephew and niece, our agency was paid by them.

He bounced back within two months of our care. Throughout those two months, his late wife' nephew tried to talk him out spending money on home care. But Mr. V. refused to give up the home care; it provided him with help and a sense of security. And after all, he said, it was his own money.

He resumed his former social life. Our social worker and nurse advised him to reduce his care from 24-hour to 10-hours shifts, which would cover all three meals, take care of shopping and cleaning and provide him with assistance on outings, such as doctor visits and social events. We hoped that he would remain safe when he was by himself during the night. This arrangement was also made to reduce the pressure that his nephew was putting on him.

For a few months the pressure subsided. Mr. V. was happy and doing well health-wise. He liked his daily routine, and developed good rapport with his aide. Unfortunately, it did not last long. Being that his nephew and niece had total control over his finances, they could manipulate Mr. V.'s. living situation. In short, Mr. V. was forced to give up his apartment, all the possessions collected over his lifetime, and move to a residential care facility. He called me every day crying and pleading to be taken out of there. I could not help him, other than to tell him to call his attorney, which turned out to be his nephew. His apartment was already gone, and essentially he had no place to go to. He had signed away all his finances and decision-making to his late wife's nephew and niece. On Mr. V.'s insistence, I tried to speak to his nephew, who basically told me to mind my own business. Mr. V. died four months later, unhappy and lonely. If anything is to be learned from Mr. V.'s experience, it is: do not rush to give someone full control over your life and finances. Always have safeguards and make iron-clad specifications as to when and what changes should be made in your life.

And make sure your attorney is not a member of your family.

Probate

Probate is a state court procedure that oversees the administration of your estate, or at least the property in your estate. There are many horror stories involving probates - delays and bureaucratic nightmares that may encourage many people to establish trusts and hold their estates out of probate. But this may not be the right move for you. An estate lawyer will be able to advise you as to your specific situation.

One should know that some banks require their own forms to be used for power of attorney, and will not accept any substitutes. Also, some states order safe deposit boxes sealed upon the tenant's death, and will not allow them to be opened until a state tax commission representative is present. Some states require a court order to open a safety deposit box that was rented in only the name of the deceased.

General Information

Although a will can be written by anyone, it is much more advisable to have a will written by an attorney. Documents that are not written in accordance with the law may be contested, or may result in higher estate taxes. It is advisable to keep the original copy with your lawyer, or if you do not have a lawyer, keep the will in a safe place that one or two people know about and is accessible to you at all times. There are many sources to find an attorney, so shop around, compare prices, and check references.

When writing a will, it is wise to state by name relatives to whom you do not wish to leave any money; consider leaving them a single dollar, so they can not contest the will by using the argument that they were omitted by error, forgetfulness, or by state of mental confusion on the writer's part when the will was written.

Other than making sure that one has established the trustees and executors, it is extremely important to empower someone to make decisions regarding health issues when the individual is unable to make those decisions for himself.

If you are like most people, you value your ability to make your own choices. You make hundreds of choices throughout any given day without giving it much thought – what to order for dinner or what to watch on TV, for example. We also make countless decisions that are much more important, such as where we will live or who our doctor will be. So it makes sense that while you are able to verbalize your wishes or make them known in any other way, you make sure that these important decisions are made clear.

If an illness renders you temporarily unconscious, unless you had made sure your loved one knew your wishes or there is a legal instrument in place for your protection, strangers with no knowledge of your wishes may have to make the decisions for you.

To protect your rights, to make your own decisions about the medical treatment you will receive, you need to do the following:

1. Complete a few simple forms to make your preferences known (a living will).
2. Select a health care agent (or proxy).
3. Make your wishes explicitly known to your health care agent, your family members and your doctor.

It does not matter if you are young old, sick or healthy, a living will and health care proxy are the ways to protect your right to make your own health care decisions. Although you may currently be in perfect health, you never know when life may throw a medical emergency your way. That is why it is important to understand the types of forms you need to have in place and how to make your wishes known under a variety of situations. The following are some of those forms:

Health Care Proxy

In this document, the individual names someone to make medical decisions for him or her, should he or she be unable to make those decisions themselves. The person you appoint may be referred to as your "health care agent," "medical power of attorney," "surrogate," or "attorney-in-fact." The document which names that person can be referred to as your "health care proxy."

The designated person must understand that she or he will need to avail themselves to the medical care providers when any medical decisions are to be made. You do not want to choose a representative who lives in another state from you, or one who is physically unable to be available to your medical team in time of need.

Leaving your health care decisions to others without any guidance from you places a great burden on your loved ones during a very traumatic time. If there is more than one opinion regarding your care from several loved ones, there is an unnecessary strain among them that is preventable. Worse yet, if there is no health proxy, a judge may appoint someone who you are not familiar with to make your medical decisions for you. That person may not know you, does not know what your values, beliefs, or preferences are.

A Durable Power of Attorney for Health Care:

This instrument gives another person of your choosing, the legal right to make medical decisions in the event that you cannot make those decisions yourself. It's very similar to the health proxy. The individual has to be fully mentally competent to sign this type of document. This document will also specify to what extent and under what conditions life support measures should be taken.

You can be the final judge as to what should or shouldn't be done to you, at the times that you are unable to clearly specify your decisions yourself. These important decisions can include mechanical intervention in cases of respiratory failure, or dialysis due to kidney failure, and if hydration and gastric feeding tubes should be inserted.

You can decide how much or how little, medical intervention you want at the last stages of your life. By doing so, you take away the decision-making from others. And with the Durable Power of Attorney for Health Care, you empower a person you trust to carry out your wishes. It is much like a will, but it deals with your medical and mental instructions, rather than with your financial ones.

There are standard forms, at no cost to you, that are available at any hospital, nursing home, and the offices of any state agency that deals with health issues. Some doctors, as well as hospitals will refuse to follow verbal instructions in less a written Durable Power of Attorney for Health Care is in place

Case # 17

My father suffered from Parkinson's disease for 14 years, the last six of which he was fully impaired by the illness. As a survivor of the Holocaust, he avoided dealing with issues involving death, so he never wrote out a will or instructed us regarding his last wishes. There would always be time for that later, he thought.

When "later" came, my mother said that my father did not want heroic measures to be implemented to unnecessarily prolong his life. I was never privy to these conversations. None of his wishes regarding the care he may require at end stages of his life were in writing.

A month before my father died, he came down with a very severe cold. It developed quickly from an upper respiratory infection to pneumonia, and we had no choice but to hospitalize him. His condition became critical and he was transferred to an intensive care unit. My whole family stayed by his side 24/7. After much argument among members of my family, he was put on a respirator; he was still conscious and could communicate by writing.

I had a young daughter and a husband at home, and a son just back from college. I worked at the time, but I put everything on hold, staying at the hospital for days at a time. My siblings did the same. As traumatic as those days were, the crisis had brought us together in our love for our father. It was clear that my father drew a great deal of support from his children and his wife being at his side.

Two weeks into his stay at the ICU, my father suffered a massive heart attack. He lapsed into unconsciousness and never regained it. The doctors kept performing all kinds of neurological test, as per our demands. But more and more grim news kept coming back: no brain activities could be detected, and their recommendation was to remove my father from life support equipment.

His organs were failing one by one, and though we knew that the only thing keeping him alive were the machines, I could not give my consent to pull the plug. He never specifically told me what he wanted me to do for him if such a situation presented itself. We all agonized, debating among ourselves, struggling with the decision with the doctors pressing us to commit to a course of action. To our eventual relief, the decision-making process was taken of our hands three days later, when God mercifully took him.

If there is a lesson in my personal story, it is this: Do not procrastinate, write down your wishes. Designate a person or persons whom you want to make those decisions when you are unable to do so yourself. It makes it easier for your own peace of mind as well as for the people who love you, allowing them to follow you requests, rather than stumbling through their own guesswork.

A Living Will

A living will is also known as a "directive to physicians," "health care declaration," or "medical directive." In this document you can list the treatments you would or would not like to be done for you, or to you, in specific situations and illnesses. This type of document will provide written record of your preferences that can guide your doctors and loved ones in caring for you, when you are too ill and unable to give them directions yourself.

In many cases, this kind of instrument will guide the measures that will be taken at the end stages of one's life. It will state how aggressive the treatments that the individual would like to be taken on his or her behalf should be. This document will state under which medical situation the patient would not like extreme measures to be instituted to sustain life.

The living will is very important for people with terminal illnesses, and advanced chronic illnesses, and should be in place before they reach those stages.

Do Not Resuscitate (DNR) order

This order may be prepared by the patient or by his or her health care proxy. It is a request not to have cardiopulmonary resuscitation performed if their heart or breathing stops. This document is only valid if it is signed by a doctor. If it is signed by a doctor it will be put then into the patient's medical chart. The DNR document is recognized by most of the states in the country.

Legal Guardianship and Conservatorship

Legal guardianship and conservatorship are legal processes for assuming control over an already incapacitated individual's affairs. A court hearing is required to grant guardianship.

This situation usually presents itself when a person has no known relatives or friends, and suddenly the person is rendered unable to care for him or herself, or make any decisions regarding financial or medical issues.

When the court is asked to intervene, usually by a social worker or protective services, the court chooses a representative, in most cases an attorney who does not know the client personally, to be responsible for the patient's affairs. Sometime a neighbor, an acquaintance, or a friend will present themselves to the court and petition for guardianship.

There are plenty of horror stories about guardians and conservators who depleted an individual's money, leaving him or her penniless, at the mercy of the government institutions, or living in poverty. It is true that if the court appoints a guardian or a conservator, they must report to the court and are answerable to the judge. But due to the overloaded schedule of the many courts around the country, in many cases, by the time the court catches on, most of the money is already gone. In all fairness, most of the appointed conservators do strive to protect the person they are appointed to protect.

While you have all your faculties, make sure you have an instrument that will protect you in the times that you are unable to make financial decisions for yourself. This will protect your assets for as long as you live. Even if the court has to appoint a guardian for you, you will still have strict written instructions for them to follow regarding your care.

I have already mentioned how important it is to keep all documents, such as the will, deed to your house, if you own one, insurance policies, health proxy, power of attorney, etc., in one place, and to let your executor or proxy know where all those documents are. Also give a copy of all these documents to your attorney, as well as to the person you designated to represent you in all matters that will affect your life and eventual death in the later years.

Chapter 10 –
Learn How to Enrich Your Life

How to Improve Quality of Life in Senior Years

If someone were to ask how we would like to see ourselves in the later years of our lives, most of us would respond: independent, healthy, and active. This is not such a far-fetched dream as had been for our parents, and even they achieved those ambitions from time to time..

The life expectancy today in the United States is 72.5 years for men, and 79.3 years for women; the average life span will increase significantly by 2050, if we learn to control the epidemic of illnesses due to overweight and decrease in physical activities in our younger population. Our society should be prepared to face the needs of the aging population that will be living much longer.

The coming years will present a need for the health care community to not only study and research ways to prolong our lives, but to find ways to make people live the extended life span in quality and fulfillment. The elderly should continue to have rich and joyful years, and not struggle with insufficient health insurance, and having to make decisions on whether to buy food or medication.

With the right educational support system, the baby boomers may be entering their senior years healthier, with better health practices, like getting sufficient sleep, exercising regularly, eating a well-balanced diet, not smoking, and having good relationships with the people in their lives. It may seem obvious, but living by those tenants really does make a difference.

A great many of the boomer generation have investments producing income, pensions, and savings that help to provide for an active and fulfilling life without financial worry. Many baby boomers are well traveled, well read, politically active, and taking part in their community activities and programs.

They will hopefully maintain and/or increase their involvement. If they continue to be active socially, take political stands, and help to form a better society for them and the seniors of the next generation, it will not only enrich their lives but also change the way the rest of the society perceives the elderly and the aging process. This generation will force improvement of existing programs, such as Social Security, Medicare and Medicaid.

The sheer voting power of 70 million people, aged 55 years and older, can practically force politicians to vote for their issues. Besides, most of the members of the Congress and Senate qualify for membership in this age group.

The employment market is also about to change. With so many people facing retirement, the market will suffer a loss of very highly experienced and productive employees. Again, although I am not an economist, I am sure the economic market can not afford it. So it easy to see that changes will be implemented to encourage workers either not to retire, or to return to the work force. Remaining fully or partially employed will be beneficial to the seniors and to the economy at large.

That shift is a win-win situation. The economy will benefit from having the additional work power, and the seniors will have the benefit of meaningful and productive years added to their lives. And the financial gain will also be an incentive.

So if you are at the stage of retiring, you should look at the possibility of continuing working, especially if it's not necessarily full time. One could live a very active life, maintaining physical activities and social activities, and continue to work.

The government should provide educational programs and guidelines, to promote better health practices. Gyms and exercise programs should be tax-deductible. Senior citizens centers that provide hot lunches for a very low fee and are subsidized by the federal government, should advocate better eating habits and educate the participants in practicing a healthy life-style.

This will promote better health in the elderly, and decrease illnesses such as high blood pressure, diabetes, heart problems, etc. Government should offer free health screening, flu shots, and blood pressure checks measured free of charge as well at senior community centers

The government should develop programs that will allow people to remain in their homes for as long as it is safe for them to do so. It should go without saying that a person would not be removed from his home for any reason other than safety issues. This is especially true for the lonely people that do not have family members involved in their lives. There should be improved programs, similar to the one existing currently, Protective Services, that can evaluate a person to see if she or he is physically and mentally safe to continue to reside in their home.

Unfortunately, many such programs today are either understaffed, or staffed with people who are inexperienced and under-trained. There should be a network to maintain the elderly in his or her home, with an oversight and connection to the community.

By now the government must recognize the fact that it is much cheaper to keep a person in his home with a home care aide, rather than to keep the same person in a nursing home. If the elderly is financially independent, and can purchase long-term care insurance, thus allowing him or her to remain home, protective services should look out for their safety, just as well as the seniors that the government pays for their care through Medicaid.

Although there are many types of insurance for long term care, and at times it is hard to navigate the field, the government should find a way to make available reasonably priced long-term insurance, which would allow seniors to remain home, living with dignity, without depleting their hard-earned savings.

A program for seniors to find centralized advisory systems should be put in place. That program will help seniors find advice on handling his or her particular needs. A social worker should be available at all times to help appropriate agencies and programs. If centralized programs are established in every city and town, there is less of a chance that some elderly person will fall through the cracks.

With such programs, the population in general becomes aware of lonely and needy persons among them. Such programs will help our seniors age with dignity. Today, this program will refer to your parent, your family member, your neighbor or friend; tomorrow, this program will provide you with the information to help you with your needs.

The baby boomers had the benefit of growing up in a time where medicine was much more available: vaccinations, antibiotics, and improved surgical procedures were the norm. New treatments for debilitating and fatal diseases have been developed. Those treatments helped to make such diseases more manageable and less deadly. New and better medications have helped to control some of the symptoms of diseases and allow for the patient to live longer and maintain their quality of life - something that was not possible in their parents' and grandparents' generation.

The development of such medications, vaccinations, and medical techniques and therapies extended the lives of many chronically and terminally ill patients. People live longer, which means that the pool of chronically ill and disabled people is growing. Unfortunately our public health system and the medical services delivery system are not adequate to provide blanket care to cover the increases. As the cost grows from year to year, the economic impact is horrendous, both for the country as a whole and on individual finances.

Such an overload on the health system will strain it, and it is urgent that the government plan for the future. It is a must that a health system is established to provide health care for the whole population, and especially for the growing pool of people 55 years and older.

The cost of medical services and insurance has been rising faster than the cost of living. The government must take control of managing the increases, by placing controls on rising prices that insurance companies can pass on to the public, and also control of what hospitals and pharmaceutical companies can charge.

What You and I Can Do

Armed with the knowledge of better health practices, we can, as a society, promote better eating habits, exercise, and promote non-smoking. Just by making the above lifestyle changes, we can improve our health and quality of life, and decrease the cost of what it takes to provide health care for such a vast population. With proper planning and foresight, we can improve our system of health management in time to withstand such a large influx of seniors.

We also need to develop better geriatric services and train professionals to deal specifically with the needs of the elderly. The local government needs to establish points of services that are easily reachable and accessible for seniors.

Centralized points of services can provide not only health care, but also educational support and nutritional support. Social services, advisory services on the benefits of Medicare and Medicaid, and other services provided by the federal government and the local government, can be made available through traditional senior centers or newly established health clinics.

A great deal of other services can be developed in these clinics as well. Social groups for community activism can be started. Lectures could be offered on topics that touch the elderly, such as sources of benefits, safe usage of medication, home health care, transportation, charities that offer free hot meals, to name a few. Many of these services can be offered at minimal or no cost.

Another source where the elderly can get services and information are from the hospitals in their own community. A great number of hospitals provide a whole range of services and programs for the benefit of the community, for old and young alike. Flu shots and advisory programs for prevention and treatment of chronic illnesses are often made available. It is always beneficial to establish a personal relationship with the staff at your neighborhood hospital.

These suggestions are not only for people who live alone, but are also for almost anyone else: any elderly person, whether healthy or sick, can benefit from these suggestions. At our website www.goldenyearsgolden.com you will find sources and resources, links, addresses, and phone numbers that can help you to find some of the existing programs that may help you in your specific case. Hopefully, in the years to come there will be a great deal more programs, as politicians and society in general will be more attuned to the needs of the seniors.

Keeping all this in mind, we as individuals need to take responsibility for our own health and practice good habits. We should eat better, practice preventive measures to protect our health, maintain good hygiene, practice good sleeping routines, exercise regularly, and, above all, be mentally stimulated.

Case # 18

Our agency took on the case of two sisters - I., who was 92 years-old, and S., who was 89 years-old. They were sweet, friendly, and shy. They had always lived together, and never married. S. became our client first after she fell and broke her hip, when her rehabilitation facility recommended us for home care. Initially we provided eight hours a day care for her, but being that I. lived there too, she also benefited from our services.

Over many visits with them, I developed a friendship with the two sisters. I found I. to be more social and outgoing. She had friends outside her home and maintained friendships for many years, long after retirement. She also went out to the theater, movies, and restaurants. S. had no friends outside her sister, and most of the time refused to go out with her sister and her fiends. She preferred to stay home alone as she did not feel comfortable socializing in a group.

When I befriended her, she seemed to open up at least a little bit. I. told me that even when they were kids, her sister was at home most of the time, and never made friends. She was frequently sick, though not with anything major - just pains here or there, multiple visits to the doctors, special diets and vitamins, etc.

Although older, I. was healthier, rambunctious, and always socializing with many friends. This pattern had followed them throughout their lives. As in their childhood, I. still felt responsible for her sister; she always made the decisions for both of them and they had always lived together.

We continued to provide home care, although it was not really needed anymore. But the sisters felt comfortable and safe having an aide there. A year later, S, then 90 years old, became ill with the flu, and she passed away a few weeks later from complications that had set in.

I was sure that S.'s death would devastate I. but she continued living in her apartment, which she had shared with her sister for 69 years. She continued to have an aide from our agency three times a week, and seemed to do well, socially and physically.

I. died six years after her sister, not of illness or old age, but in a tragic accident, hit by a speeding taxi while crossing the street. She suffered massive injuries which left her paralyzed. I visited I. in the hospital, and knew that the will to live had left her. She died peacefully a few days later. I. lived 99 years, a full life, a rich life. She never had a husband or children, yet she was happy and her life was full of people, friends, and coworkers. Even the aides that took care of her had become her friends.

In recent years, numerous studies have been conducted on the subject of what happiness is, and how social interaction affects our well-being and our health. The difference between I.'s and S.'s approaches to life and socialization supports the old saying that no man should be an island.

So, if you are taking care of a parent, relative, or a friend, it is important that you take into account the social needs of that person. Check if there are any senior citizen centers in the neighborhood, and what kind of activities they provide. Most of the senior citizen centers will provide transportation to and from activities.

In some of the centers you may find a rich range of activities, such as physical exercise, art, dancing and field trips. It is important to make sure that the senior's doctor approves him or her for these activities, and if there are any restrictions, the center should be made aware of them.

If the person you are taking care of is used to socializing a great deal, encourage him or her to continue to maintain friendly relations with their friends and neighbors, and open their home, making it pleasant to visitors.

Another aspect that we need to consider when caring for our parent or relative is their self-image - how they feel about themselves. It would be advisable to leave as much of the everyday decision-making to them, regarding everyday tasks. The person should decide what he or she wants to wear, or whether to shower or bathe upon rising in the morning or at night, before going to sleep. Some sense of control should be left to them for as long as possible.

The most important thing for the elderly is to maintain an active and stimulating life. Mental abilities can be maintained for a long time, by encouraging the person to stimulate his or her brain with puzzles, mental exercises, reading, and social interaction with others. Without mental stimulation, the person's mental abilities will slowly decrease just as their muscles atrophy without physical activity.

Stimulate the elderly and their environment with visual and audio as well as physical stimulation. An environment full of music, social contact, exchanges of pictures, access to books with large lettering, if needed, as well as trips to shopping and movie theaters will be great for mental stimulation and an improved quality of life for the elderly.

Physical activities should be encouraged. Even the slightest physical activities, such as repetitious movement, will benefit the elderly, bringing blood to the brain and with it oxygen, for improved mental abilities. Most physical activities result in huge benefits. Walking strengthens the heart and the cardiovascular system, and it reduces the risk of heart disease.

Exercise need not to be long in duration - just three to four times a week and only 15 to 20 minutes per session can be extremely beneficial to the elderly. One needs to clear any regimen with their personal doctor, what physical activities they can do and can not do.

The following benefits can be derived from physical activities by seniors, or for that matter, by anybody:

- Reverse bone loss and stops bone depletion.

- Improves symptoms of chronic diseases, such as back pain, ambulation difficulties, etc.

- People with disabilities benefit exercising.

- Relieves depression.

- Improves sleep, regardless of the actual amount of time spent exercising.

- Physical activities improve appetite, increases alertness, sharpness, and response time.

- Lowers the risk of falls and injury, if done properly and according to doctor's instruction. Also improves mobility strength and circulation.

- Visibly improves skin tone for women.

- If done regularly, improves the function of bladder and bowel system.

- In general, improves the working of the liver, pancreases, and other organs, as well as strengthens muscles, tendons, and ligaments.

There is no question that physical activities are beneficial to us all, we just need to be attuned to our bodies, and not do harm to ourselves while exercising. We also need to start slowly, and build it up gradually giving our muscles time to adapt to the strain.

The best scenario would be to encourage seniors partake in physical activities in senior citizen centers or local Ys; they will benefit doubly, between the actual physical activity and the social interaction. Group exercise provides the participants with health benefits, as well as mental benefits, and may even bring new friendships to the senior's life. Research also shows who seniors that have good relationships with members of their family do much better mentally in the later years of their lives.

Besides providing a mentally stimulating environment, we should also pay attention to the physical condition of the senior. Although it is highly likely that most of us will develop some chronic illness in our later years, it is possible to diminish the effects on our everyday lives.

When I first heard the expression, "today's sixties are yesterday's forties," it sounded so appropriate. The 60-year old seniors of today feel youthful, energized, and, for the most part, very active in their society.

But when seniors reach a more advanced age, when one's health is not at its best, society needs to be prepared to provide the care they need, paid for privately, through national health coverage, or a combination of the two. We are bombarded by the media with news about the epidemics of different factors that affect our health, and have become or will become an issue to our society. One of these epidemics we hear a great deal about today is obesity.

Statistically, the number of Americans who are developing diabetes, high blood pressure, and high cholesterol, are growing rapidly. It is predicted that for the first time, our children are projected to live a shorter life span than their parents, due to their lifestyle. The children of today have unhealthy eating habits, basing their diet on fast food that promotes diabetes and high blood pressure.

Compounding that trend is the sedentary lifestyle that our children lead today. They spend most of the after-school hours in front of their television sets, or in front of their computers. Their physical activities have decreased, suggesting they will become adults with greater physical problems.

The following elements play a great deal in our health and well-being:

Take Care of Yourself

NUTRITION

We can discuss this issue of importance to the aging population in a general way. We all know that food is the fuel of life, but it can also be a cause of health problems, such as high blood pressure, diabetes, and heart disease, if the wrong foods are regularly eaten.

In the post-World War II era, as a new society developed, prosperity settled in slowly. Food became plentiful and cheep. Anyone could walk into a supermarket and buy whatever he or she desired. Over the years food production increased, delivering to the consumer a wide variety of processed food. Yet in processing the food for a long shelf-life, the tradeoff was that many nutrients have been lost. As Americans focus on how food tastes or how much it costs, the nutritional value of what we consume is often overlooked and forgotten.

Most fast foods available to us are high in fats, sugar, and preservatives. By eating a lot of carbohydrates, mostly processed and refined, we exposed ourselves to many diseases, such as type 2 diabetes. This is changing somewhat now that we are more knowledgeable about proper nutrition, and more of us are making better choices as to what and how much we eat. There are thousands of books that cover the topic of nutrition, and how it relates to our health, but of course only a few of us will actually read up on the subject in depth. The Internet also offers plenty of material on the subject. Of course people in their seventies and older, may not have a computer, so their information has to come from other sources.

Your doctor is a great source of knowledge regarding your nutrition, and how it relates to you and your needs. He or she will advise you what your diet should be, what combination of foods should be eaten together, or should be avoided entirely. Dieticians are available, and most insurance plans will cover the cost of a visit. Unfortunately, 47 million Americans have no health insurance, and therefore no access to consultations with doctors or dieticians who can instruct on healthy and appropriate eating habits.

Uninsured Americans often receive their medical care in an emergency room. The care is provided fast and is not on a very personal basis, and in all likelihood it does not include an education in proper nutrition. Maybe in the coming years, when every American, young and old, is provided health coverage, nutritional education will be part of that universal coverage.

When we consider the needs of the elderly, the priority of proper nutrition is even more important. In my work I have encountered many elderly people who were malnourished, or had out-of-control diabetes, from inappropriate diet. For the elderly, it is often difficult to correct the damages caused by poor nutrition.

Every client served by our agency was evaluated for their nutritional needs by their doctor with the support of a nutritionist, in order to help them to regain their health or improve their health. All meals were prepared based on direct instruction of the doctor and nutritionist. And over time one could see a difference in the patients, directly due to the care and good nutrition.

When seniors are in a nursing home, assisted living facility, or residential care facility, their diets are controlled and geared to their health issues, and their food is prepared to promote improvement in their health. Whatever is needed for their good health is, or should be, provided. But an elderly person living in his or her own home alone, with minimal or no support system, may be affected by poor nutrition.

The ideal scenario for the future is proper support and instruction for the elderly, including free-of-charge services of a dietician trained in geriatric needs. A dietician would educate the elderly in making the right food choices and preparation of nutritious foods, as well as the development of nutritious meal plan. Now that the senior population is increasing, it is also time for the food companies to consider the aging population when packaging foods. Nutritional contents should be listed clearly, in bold letters, so the elderly with impaired vision can read them. More products should be sodium-free for the benefit of the elderly. We all could use less sodium in our diets, regardless of our health status.

Supermarkets should stock products to attract seniors, by placing many of the products on middle shelves, so the seniors need not reach high, nor bend down to reach for the product. With the physical limitations of the elderly in mind, changes could be made to ease shopping for seniors. Deliveries, free of charge, and special pricing should be made afforded to the elderly.

Combining poor diets with sedentary lifestyles has caused us to become an overweight society; and as a result we are suffering many underlying illnesses. This may affect the elderly in a more devastating way. So it is essential that we combine nutritious diet with physical activities, with the direction and permission from the seniors' doctors. No matter how minimal the activity may be, it will be beneficial to the senior.

Scientists are finding that what we eat can make us either sick or healthy. There are many studies that show that eating a nutritious diet can keep you healthy and allow you to live longer. Correlations between certain foods and certain cancers have been studied; scientists are also finding that some foods are helpful with easing pain, such as arthritis.

In very general terms, you should eat as healthy as possible. You should include in your diet plenty of fruits and vegetables. And if you're not restricted by your doctor, those can be eaten either raw or cooked. Evidence shows green vegetables, such as spinach, endives, broccoli, and beans of all sorts, and foods high in vitamin B-12 can help keep our cognitive abilities high. Nuts are also very nutritious, assuming you are not allergic to them. You should consume healthy oils, such as olive oil and canola oil. Decrease the amount of red meat in your diet, and increase the amount of fish. You should eat whole grain breads, pasta, and cereal; whole grains are rich in fiber, which is beneficial to your heart.

Ask your doctor or dietician for a diet plan that is appropriate for you to maintain a healthy body, and help you enjoy your life to the fullest.

One of the books that I found very useful for understanding of the benefits of proper nutrition, as well as physical activities, was Dr. Andrew Weil's *Healthy Aging*. There are hundreds of books on the subject of nutrition geared toward the elderly; pick one most suitable for you.

Case # 19

One of the more challenging cases we had in our agency was a client who selected our agency from the Yellow Pages. Ms. A. was a woman in her mid fifties, who behaved like a stubborn child most of the time.

By the time we started to provide home care for Ms. A. she had major health problems, most of which were exasperated by her behavior, which bordered on suicidal tendencies. Among her illnesses, she had uncontrolled diabetes, which had already cost her a leg. She was bound to a wheelchair, which she used on the rare occasion she ventured out of her home. She stayed in her bed for days, refusing to bathe, eat at the table, or change clothing.

As it is our practice, we require the client to provide us with the name of his or her doctors, who normally advises us as to patient's medical status, and to the care we should provide. Based on this channel of communication, we develop a plan of care, and directed our aide as to her appointed tasks at the patient's home.

But we had a very difficult time obtaining information from Ms. A. She refused to give us the doctor's information, contending that she was fully capable of handling her own health issues. She ordered her medication from her doctor, as well as from her pharmacist, without involving the visiting nurse or the aide from our agency.

We finally contacted Ms. A's doctor, by having the aide asking the receptionist for doctor's name and phone number, while escorting Ms. A. on a visit to that doctor.

The aide called in the information to the agency, and one of our nurses rushed over to the doctor's office, insisting to see the doctor, while Ms. A. was still in the office. She explained the situation to the doctor, and asked him, in front of Ms A, to help us to develop an appropriate plan of care for her. Put on the spot, Ms. A. relented and allowed the doctor to guide us and help us to take care of her in the most beneficial way.

The doctor said the most important issue in her health situation was control her sugar levels. This would require setting up an appropriate dietary plan, under the direction of a dietician specializing in diabetic diets. Ms. A. agreed that she would cooperate with our staff, let the aide shop and prepare food, and follow a strict diet. The doctor said: "As I said a million times before, you're killing yourself by continuing to eat the way you do, by not taking your medications as instructed, and by being totally inactive. Please let the people from the agency help you." She promised to do so.

Ms. A. also agreed to become more physically active, working out with a physical therapist, and going out daily if the weather permitted. She also agreed to daily bathes and changes of clothing.

We had high hopes, now that we knew how to help Ms. A. With the guidance of the dietician, our aide prepared daily meals that aimed to reduce sugar levels and add nutritionally balance. Very quickly, this became a very agitating issue for the patient. She refused to eat the meals that were prepared for her, and continued her old habits of ordering in food that were loaded with sugars, that were detrimental to her health.

Within days she was back to her old routine, refusing to take daily baths, or to get out of bed, and continued to order unhealthy foods over the phone - inappropriate foods in inappropriate sizes, like an entire pizza pie that she would order and polish off herself at midnight.

She was always abusive with the people who worked for her, but the abuse had increased. Aides began to refuse to work for her. I went over to speak to her; I tried to explain to Ms. A. that we cannot work in a situation where the patient disregards all of the instructions given by her doctor, the dietician, and the nurse. We are there to help, but the patient needs to want to accept that help and do their part.

While I was doing my best to make Ms. A. understand how serious her health problems were, she pulled out a large chocolate from under her pillow, unwrapped it, and ate the whole chocolate there in front of me without a blink of an eye. I just sat there for a few minutes, completely in shock; I just could not understand how an intelligent person could undermine their own health like that.

Right then and there, I informed Ms. A. that we would have to ask her to seek home care from another agency. She did not think that we actually would give up on such a "lucrative case" as she referred to herself. But we decided that we could not in all good conscience continue a case that we could not help, and stand by and watch her do all the things that the professional people around her instructed her not to do.

Ms. A. moved on to another agency, she continued the same pattern of behavior and her health rapidly deteriorated. Seven months after she switched to another agency for her care, her kidneys failed her and by the end of the year she died. She was only 56 at the time of her death.

I cannot stop thinking that her death could have been avoided.

The story of Ms. A. could be a lesson to all of us, to stress the importance of following doctor's instructions, and to maintain an active and healthy lifestyle.

Taking care of yourself

SLEEP

Getting enough sleep is also essential for one's good health. The amounts of hours one needs can vary for each of us. Some of us will need eight hours, and others can function quite well on six hours of sleep.

From different studies, it appears that people who sleep for six hours without interruption, benefit more than the person who sleeps eight hours with interruptions. The best advice I have received from a doctor, is try to teach your body to nap - half an hour, an hour, however much time you can spare. The nap will rejuvenate you and give you a boost of energy.

As we age, our sleep patterns change. Sleep is important throughout human life, and people who sleep longer with fewer interruptions tend to be healthier and recuperate faster from bouts of illnesses and surgery. Studies show that people who nap regularly tend to maintain higher mental capacity then people who do not nap.

Many of us in this country have sleeping problems, some more than others. Many of us rely on medications to help us fall asleep, or to maintain a significant amount of sleep. There are many practices that can aid us with establishing and maintaining beneficial and healthy patterns of sleep.

It's advisable to learn your personal sleeping habits. Do you get sleepy at a particular time in the evening? Do you tend to eat late at night? Do you drink a great deal before going to sleep? Will you continue to watch television, or read a book, in spite of feeling sleepy? Do you watch television while in bed? All those things impact your sleep. Once you determine your patterns of sleep, you may conclude what interferes with a good night of sleep. Some of the things can easily be corrected, and a noticeable improvement can result when changes are made.

Let's talk about some of the items that undermine a good and refreshing sleep:

a. Eating a full meal or even small snacks can affect your sleep. It is best not to eat at least two or three hours before going to sleep.

b. Watching television, or reading a book in a room other then the bedroom should be done in a sitting position. The bedroom should be designated for sleeping.

c. Try to maintain regular hours for sleeping. Our body is built on habits and routines. If you go to sleep regularly at about 10 pm, your body will adjust to this time. But if you change the time you go to sleep every evening, you throw off your biological clock, confusing your body.

d. If you need to get up during the night, try not turn on many lights, you may want to keep a small night light for such occasions. The brighter the light, the more awake you become, and the harder it will be to fall asleep again.

e. Some people will make a habit of drinking warm milk with a teaspoon of honey before retiring for the night. It's an old remedy, but some people swear by it.

f. Maintain room temperature that is suitable to you, so you are not too cold or too hot. That it is, if you can control it. Most people will sleep better if the temperature is just few degrees lower.

g. If you're having trouble falling asleep, just relax, close your eyes, and rest. This may lead you to eventually fall asleep.

h. Make sure to spend a few hours outside, to benefit from direct sunlight. An hour or two outdoors will benefit you in general and promote better sleep patterns.

As a child I always thought that napping was for babies. But now I know better. If you can establish a routine, where you regularly take an hour or two hour nap in the afternoon, you will add hours of sleep and eliminate sleep deficiencies. If your daily schedule permits it, you will be surprised how easy it is to get into the habit of napping, and how great the benefit is for your body.

The benefits from napping are not only physical, they are also mental. You will find that you are energetic and easily mentally stimulated when you are rested. Your disposition also improves when you body is rested. Napping time does not have to be long, even 30 minutes proves quite refreshing.

The whole idea of resting means that you are doing absolutely nothing. That is not as easy a task as it sounds. We are bombarded with stimuli at all times. It is hard to disconnect fully and try to relax. But it is a learned ability, and if repeated regularly, it will become second nature. So make sure you factor in a time to rest on a regular basis.

It is essential that we get enough sleep; when we are deprived of it we open ourselves to all kinds of trouble. Over time lack of sleep decreases our mental effectiveness and promotes many illnesses. As we age, as mentioned before, our pattern of sleep changes. We sleep less, not as deeply, and we wake up one to two times per night. So it is up to you to develop a good routine of sleep, by minimizing the amount of stimulation at the time you go to sleep.

STRESS

One of the factors that interfere with our ability to relax and sleep well is stress. We all know that life is stressful, it always has been, and in all likelihood, always will be. But stress plays out differently for each of us, affects us all differently. Nonetheless, we should learn how to cope with our stress, and try to minimize it. Studies show that stress affects us physically, and it has a greater effect on the elderly, who have more difficulties coping with it. The greater the stress and the longer you live with it, the greater the damage it does to you.

So the initial step is to pinpoint the source of your stress. If at all possible, when you identify what it is that causes your stress, try to remove that cause, or at least reduce it. Many people use different relaxation techniques, such as meditation or yoga. I find that using daily physical exercise helps me to relax and reduce stress. All such activities, whichever ones you choose for your reduction of stress, should be cleared with your doctor.

Promoting health has not been a high priority on our national agenda. Most of us in this country live with a constant worry that we will suddenly lose our health insurance coverage, due to some catastrophic illness or to the inability to pay for the ever-increasing cost of insurance. That too, increases our stress level.

One of the things missing in our health care system is psychological support geared to the elderly. Many family doctors will be happy to prescribe some psychotropic medication upon diagnosis of depression, but rarely is the patient evaluated by a psychiatrist to determine the cause. Many seniors come from a generation that looked upon psychiatric treatment in a very negative way.

Stress and depression should be diagnosed and treated promptly in the elderly; if untreated, it is likely to cost the health care system much more when complications arise. In many cases, it is too late when we notice that the elderly are stressed or depressed, when their mental behavior has changed, when they have noticeably lost weight and become malnourished, have withdrawn from society, or develop other illnesses.

Education of the caregivers includes detection, and the treatment of stress and depression in the elderly in the early stages. Psychiatric care should be available to the elderly, if needed, through Medicare at little or no cost. The cost of the medications to treat psychiatric problems should also fully be covered by Medicare.

When you think about it, aging is not an easy thing to accept. You're getting older and your body is slowly failing you. It wasn't that long ago that you were independent, providing a shoulder that others leaned on and suddenly you need to depend on others for the simplest of tasks. So it's no wonder you get depressed. And many of us do not have someone close, a relative or a friend, to reassure, protect, and look out for us, leading to more insecurities and depression.

Much of the stress that we experience through life involves financial issues – how we will provide for ourselves and our kids, the state economy, the cost of college, one's job, and hundreds other worries. But when we are younger, we are better able to deal with stress. There are options available to us; we have choices that we can make, and that in itself reduces stress. When we age, we have fewer choices, we worry more, and therefore we experience more stress.

If you notice that your parent is stressed, the causes may sometimes look trivial to you, but it is not so much the cause of the stress, rather the stress itself that can harm them. So it is essential that you deal with the stress, and not disregard it.

Prolonged bouts of stress will contribute to development of illnesses or make the illness they already have much worse. So it is very important that your or your parent's personal physician be informed about the stress that you or your parent is experiencing. The physician may check for underlying reasons for the stress, and if there is a medical reason, he or she may recommend either medication or psychological treatment.

Society can not alleviate all the causes of stresses from our elderly but some of the causes can be eliminated. Worries like how much their health needs will be covered, or if their medication will be available to them, should be avoidable.

Seniors need assurance that their basic needs are covered, such as their residential situation - whether home care, nursing home care, or any residential situation in between. You need to reassure and encourage them to feel useful and wanted; no one wants to feel like they are a burden to their children, which is big stress inducer.

Encourage physical activity, because exercise is a great stress reducer. Social interaction also promotes stress reduction. Healthier and happier people tend to be less stressed. I hope you and you loved one will be happy, healthy, and stress free. But if stress is part of your life, do not disregard it, make sure that you deal with it, and try to reduce it.

PHYSICAL ACTIVITIES

It is a known fact, that the maintenance of healthy aging is based greatly on healthy eating habits and a very active life, physically and mentally. A well-developed physical routine, with the approval of your physician, is essential in maintaining good health.

Most elderly who have maintained their good health into the later years of their lives will tell you that besides the good genes that they may have been blessed with, they had healthy eating habits and a lifetime of running, walking, dancing, and playing golf or tennis, practicing yoga, or filled with other physical activities.

As we get older, all activities should be monitored and approved by a doctor, as I have hammered home before. One should do all physical activities in moderation. I regret to say that I too have discovered the benefits of physical activities rather late in my life, and had to build up my routines slowly. I felt guilty for not exercising, and I did know that I should be doing the exercise for my own health. Slowly, over several months, I developed a routine of going to a gym four to five times a week, and following a routine outlined for me by a physical instructor who designed the routine based on my doctor's recommendation and my personal physical needs.

I admit that I still do not particularly care for the actual exercise, but my body feels wonderful afterwards, and this makes me want to go the next day. Many people that I have interviewed for this book have told me that after getting themselves into shape, their doctors found that they needed lower doses of medication for diseases such as diabetes and high blood pressure, and at times were removed from medication totally.

There most likely is a neighborhood gym, senior citizen center, Y or community center that has exercise classes suited for the elderly. Some of them may be offer them free of charge, or for a very minimal fee.

Participating in those programs may have more than just physical benefits, but also mental and emotional ones. Additionally there are many social benefits in group exercise.

In many of the senior citizens centers you can find mentally stimulating activities. The more activities your loved one gets involved in, the longer he or she will maintain their mental faculties; studies show that seniors who interact socially and fill their life with a stimulating routines, mentally and physically, remain healthier and mentally alert much longer. Seniors that are sedentary and who are loners tend to fare much worse.

There is no question that in the coming years, with the increasing number of seniors in society, the business community will concentrate on the vast possibilities and profit gains centered on seniors' needs. It is fair to assume that there will many more facilities developed to provide such programs. The business community will see the marketing possibilities involved in devising tools and activities to promote mental and physical stimulation. Accessibility of programs provided to the elderly, with their doctors' approval, will be beneficial to them, promoting good mental and physical health.

Hundreds of studies have been done to prove that together, with good nutrition, rest, and preventive medical care, physical activity will improve the overall health status of the person practicing it. We've all heard personal stories of people who after starting a good exercise regimen, have reduced their weight and regulated their blood pressure, removing the need for high blood pressure medication. The same holds true for people diagnosed with diabetes; with the same regimen they ended up no longer needing to take medication to regulate their sugar levels.

Now that I have been going to the YMCA on a regular basis, I have realized what a wonderful place it is for its members. There are so many senior citizens that come there on a regular basis. Many programs are geared for them, such as swimming, aquatic aerobics for the ones with joint problems. They offer yoga, aerobics, ballroom dancing, and many other programs for the seniors.

YMCA and YMHA are very much community oriented. There are lectures on varied topics, something to interest everyone. I see groups of seniors sitting together and socializing and establishing friendships. One senior said to me, "coming here is the best part of my day." The cost is set several levels, based on what members can afford. If one cannot pay at all, there are subsidies available, allowing everyone to become a member.

In the chapter that discusses the future of our health system and improving the quality of our later years, I mentioned that a centralized point of services should be established in which information, vaccinations, social work advisory stations, etc., could be provided for the elderly. Such places as our YMCA come close to what those centers should be. Many of the new retirement communities, residential facilities, and senior citizen centers have gyms, such as pools, equipment, or classes that are geared to the seniors.

In all gyms you will find personnel who specialize in exercise activities geared to the elderly, and all their limitations. When I spoke with some of the personnel in gyms, they all said that they are seeing older clients, and thus they are starting to plan and develop special programs for them.

Because the senior population has a higher risk for diseases such as high blood pressure, diabetes, back or other skeletal problems, and although exercise is very beneficial to them, the instructors should have the knowledge as to what exercises they can or can not do. It is advisable to have a standard rule that the client, regardless of age, bring a form from his or her physician, as to what limitation they have and clearing them for physical activity. The physicians' instructions should be the guide for developing an exercise plan for the each individual.

Exercise can be extremely beneficial to the senior; it can slow down the process of aging, and help to maintain the energy and vitality that otherwise would not be there. But you have to remember that the age factor makes us more vulnerable to injury, so caution should be exercised at all times.

Dr. Walter Bortz, author of the books "Dare to Be 100" and "Living Longer for Dummies," said quite eloquently, "Fitness for young people is an option; fitness for old people is an imperative." We should therefore make it available to all seniors. Part of the investment society can make for its elders, is to provide such facilities free of charge, staffed by personnel that is trained to provide services and instructions for the seniors. It pays for itself by lowering health care costs in the long run.

Regular physical activity will help seniors maintain their physical strength and allow them to have more energy and hence be more independent. This is true for younger people too. Exercise on a regular basis is also known to decrease depression and help fight diseases such as diabetes, heart disease, and cancer.

Exercise routines do not have to be very elaborate to have a positive effect. An elderly person can be encouraged to start slowly, with just walks around the neighborhood. Starting with five-minute walks, one can then slowly increase them to 10 minutes, and then to longer increments over time. Walking for ten or fifteen minutes a few times a week will do a great deal of good for you. If you can develop this routine with another person, it will help you maintain the routine over time as well as provide socialization.

Not only is walking a good exercise, it is free. One does not need membership to expensive facilities, a fixed schedule, or instructions; all one needs is the willingness to go outside and start walking. Just put one foot in front of the other. The walker is the one who sets the tempo of the walk, when and where it will take place.

If the senior has limited ambulation and walking is not an option, exercises from a sitting position can be developed. Simple exercises using one's limbs keep one's muscles toned and functioning.

When I worked in nursing homes years ago, we set up exercise sessions where the seniors sat in either wheelchairs or chairs in a circle, lifting their arms or legs to the extent they could, accompanied by music or singing to make it more fun. The key is movement. The more movement, the better. It was always kept at each individual's own pace.

In the last 30 to 40 years, we have come to understand more and more of the impact that physical activity has on our health. Every doctor you visit will encourage you to exercise and be more active. Any physical activity is beneficial, but should first be approved by a doctor.

I personally was never eager to exercise on a regular basis. I occasionally enjoyed a game of tennis, but as I aged, I noticed that my game slowed down, and finally it stopped after an injury to my knee and lower back. With high blood pressure and borderline sugar numbers, I was under constant pressure from my doctor to start a regular regimen of physical activities. I knew I had to start taking appropriate steps, I wrote down all the reasons for starting regular exercise. I visited a physical therapist, and worked out a routine suitable to my age and health condition. What I have found useful to motivate me to persistently maintain my routine, was keep a visible list of reasons for the importance of the physical activities I was doing, and mark each day on the calendar what exercises I had done that day.

The best news came on the day when I found out my blood pressure medication was cut in half. So, my advice would be to do whatever works for you to motivate yourself, to become active to the level of your ability, and with the approval of your doctor.

As the number of seniors increases, it will benefit our government to provide, whether through health insurance companies or through Medicare, physical activities available to everyone through all senior citizen centers or other public facilities free of charge. As I have mentioned before, all these programs can be offered through existing facilities, such as the one mentioned throughout this chapter, or through churches, synagogues, outpatient clinics, and school facilities. This will allow exercise programs in each neighborhood, to be in close proximity to seniors' places of residence.

It is much cheaper to pay for physical activity programs than for treatments of illnesses that become chronic, and long-term treatments that are very costly. I think we have reached a time that it is wise to change the old ways of thinking that we have practiced up to now in our health system. Making good physical activities programs available, free-of-charge or with minimal charge, to all of us will promote good health to an active and energetic population and will decrease exuberant costs in the future.

EMOTIONAL WELL-BEING

Although all of us have emotional needs, and age seems to factor in them at all stages, the emotional needs of the elderly tend to be more complex, commanded by the dependency and loss of independence that become part of their lives.

We all need positive reinforcement in our daily lives, be it in school, at work or in our homes, when we are children or as adults, as spouses and as parents. Most of us have the need to receive positive feedback as to how well we are doing, for whatever we are doing. When we get older, our emotional needs are different. We want to know that we still matter, that we count. We need to know that our opinion is valued, respected, and always taken into account. When you deal with seniors, always be tuned in to their emotional needs, especially if those affect their well-being and their daily quality of life. When you notice a problem, you should seek out professional help for them.

We often make common mistake in the way we interact with our parents when they become older. I deal more extensively with the role reversal syndrome in the chapter on role reversal, but even if the needs in your specific situation are such that they require you to take over the role of caring for and making decisions for your parent or the senior, they should not feel that you're treating him or her as a child.

Although my mother is dependent on me and my brothers for all decision-making regarding her financial and medical issues, she still demands to be in the loop, and we run everything by her, even if it sometimes takes repeating. And even though she usually responds by saying "You know best what should be done," it does make her feel that things are not decided for her, but with her.

Another source of emotional ups and downs can be health issues. Once an illness, acute, chronic, or even one of short duration that has a very good prognosis of recovery, is diagnosed, seniors can understandably respond very emotionally. They worry how such an illness will affect them in the future. They worry about being sick, about not recovering quickly, or ever fully recovering. And they worry if the illness will make them change their lives - if their illness will make them totally dependent on their children, or caregivers.

For example, if a senior has broken a hip and his or her ambulation is affected, whether temporarily or permanently, can you see what it may do to them emotionally?

The psychological and mental status of the patient will affect the rate and speed of recovery, and at times will determine if the patient will return to what his or her functional status was before the injury.

Although most of the medical staff dealing with the geriatric population is aware of the emotional needs that this particular population has, not all are trained to deal with the problems at hand. With such a large number of seniors coming into the pool of the population, as more baby boomers reach that age group in the next ten years, we should make sure that in addition to their medical and health needs, their mental and emotional needs will be provided for when necessary.

Where the system is currently lacking, we need to encourage family and friends to step in and provide emotional support for their loved ones, and to be on the lookout for signs of depression and emotional issues. If signs of depression are noticed by the family member or caregiver, they need to inform the patient's doctor and seek out a professional mental health therapist.

Besides suffering from depression, the elderly may also suffer from anxiety. Some people worry more than needed, and the anxiety bouts follow them throughout life. At times anxiety grows in people's later years, and begins to affect their everyday life. The elderly suffering from anxiety tend to become suspicious and mistrusting of the people around them.

People suffering from anxiety can also exhibit symptoms such as restlessness, irritability, difficulty to sleeping, difficulty in concentrating on tasks. They can be extremely vigilant and edgy. They constantly worry about financial matters and about being ill. Among other symptoms exhibited by elderly with anxiety are panic disorders, compulsive behavior, fear of closed places, and other phobias.

Anxiety, like other mental disorders, can be related to medications, or certain types of physical illnesses. When such symptoms are obvious, help should be offered to the senior by his or her doctor through therapy or medication. Treatment may include relaxation techniques. The support of family and friends is extremely important to reduce anxiety in the elderly.

Some doctors, as well as family members, can be dismissive of the anxiety issues that an elderly person is experiencing, but it should be taken with the utmost of seriousness because it is very real to the individual experiencing it, and it affects him or her both physically and mentally.

THE POWER OF MEDITATION AND PRAYER

Throughout the years of working with the elderly and the ill, I have seen the importance of the power of prayer and meditation. I have seen very ill people, with pain making even the smallest of movement extremely difficult and who could barely breathe, whose strong belief in God, the prayer brought such tranquility to them. I am envious of the strength of their faith.

Many studies have been done on the subject of the power of faith and prayer; most suggest that people who practice the belief and prayer do better. I have seen patients with strong belief in nursing homes cope with their illness much better than patients that were despondent and gave up on the possibility of getting better.

Theories of different types of meditation suggest that people who meditate on a regular basis, fare better with illnesses, and get better sooner, than people who do not meditate. From my own experience, which is not based on scientific research, I have seen what strong faith and the power of prayer have done for very ill people.

If one has the support of their church, synagogue, mosque, or any other form of religious institution, they tend to do better with dealing with the hardships that life puts before them. People interacting in group prayers, and meditation sessions tend to be more social and less isolated. Those people tend to be more able to reach out to others for help, and more receptive to accept help when it is offered to them.

Almost all nursing homes provide religious services and programs on a regular basis, weekly, or even more frequently. There are many residents in nursing homes who are very involved in those religious activities, setting up and running the services if a clergy member is not available. When asked what they get out of it, the residents always said that it was very fulfilling and enriching for them to do those tasks.

I look at prayer as having a conversation with God or some higher power, whatever the individual's personal beliefs. It is a way to release stress, to ease burdens, in a very unconditional way. Most of us are familiar with prayers since our childhood. Some of us pray and worship our religion throughout life. Others come back to religion and praying in their later years and find solace in the process.

I had clients who, when faced with terminal illness, turned to faith for strength, each praying and worshipping in his or her own way. It brought them comfort and strength in dealing with their illness.

Although it has been around for thousands of years, meditation is much less practiced by the elderly. This may change in the years to come. With all the baby boomer becoming senior citizens, we are likely to see meditation gaining steam. First, many of the baby boomers practiced yoga and meditation throughout their younger years and are likely to continue this practice. Second, meditating does not need to be linked to religion. One does not need special equipment, or to belong to a gym; you can sit down on the floor, in your bed, on a chair, or on a sofa. You can sit in your home, in your garden, or in a park. Just clear your head of all troublesome thoughts, and by repeating a simple word, humming, or relaxing, you clear your mind of all that is troubling you.

When I decided to try meditation, I was instructed to clear my mind of all thoughts that could disrupt my concentration, to relax each muscle, limb by limb, while sitting comfortably and not necessarily in any particular position. Concentrating on one part of my body and repeating one word slowly, until my body relaxed. Total relaxation engulfed me and with it a sense of peacefulness.

Initially it was hard for me to develop a routine of total relaxation. My mind kept returning to issues that troubled me, to tasks that I needed to deal with after finishing my meditating. But by doing it repeatedly, I finally got the hang of it. And surprisingly, I found it very relaxing. The first thing I noticed after regularly devoting 20 minutes of meditating daily, was that my blood pressure dropped significantly, so much so that my doctor decreased my blood pressure medication by half.

I also noticed after practicing meditation regularly that I was much more relaxed. Things that used to irritate me and cause me much distress do not have the same effect on me anymore. My energy level also increased, while my stress level noticeably decreased - I am sure that it was a direct outcome of the meditation.

Nursing homes, senior citizen center, assisted living facilities, retirement communities, and residential care facilities all should develop regular programs of meditation geared to the physical limitations of the elderly. They may not be able to sit on the floor and would therefore require comfortable chairs or sofas where they can sit safely. The lighting should also be comfortable for the seniors, not too high or sharp, and not too dark, so if someone gets up and leaves the room, he or she will not trip and fall.

So remember, meditation does not require special physical abilities, instructions are very simple to follow, and it does not require special equipment, or expensive membership clubs. It is easy to instruct, and easy to participate in a meditation session. The elderly can take part in meditation session even if they are disabled, or whether or not they are ambulatory, or whether they have visual, hearing, or speech impairments. We all can do it and benefit from it.

There are many techniques to practice meditation and you can pick the one that is suited for you, and with which you feel comfortable.

Reinventing Retirement

Despite the fact that not every one of us is covered by health insurance and has access to medical care and preventive medical care, we are enjoying greater longevity than our grandparents did. The fact is that we are living longer. That is the one of the greatest achievements of our time. A child born today can expect to live 30 years longer than a child born in the beginning of last century, although these gains are in danger due to the epidemic of obesity and diabetes that are sweeping our nation.

This longevity will define the way we see, plan, and live our retirement. It is clear that in preparation for retirement, baby boomers will ponder as to how they will spend the next 30 or 40 years of their life.

Retirement is a fairly new idea – just over a half century ago, people did not retire. Most people worked until they died, or became ill and unable to continue working. Most had to continue working, and were unable to stop working even in their seventies due to financial needs.

Nowadays, we still are active at retirement age and not rushing to join the ranks of retirees. Many people 65 and older are choosing to continue to work, even after reaching retirement age. We are healthier, we live longer, and many of us are not ready to stop working, even if we can afford to retire financially.

For those who do choose to retire, relatively new health and economic changes, as well as the Social Security and Medicare programs, have allowed us to retire when we still fairly healthy and young enough to continue to enjoy life and maintain productivity.

Most Americans do not engage in hard physical labor as our parents did. With the labor laws that were developed to protect workers, we have a reasonable work day, usually not exceeding eight hours. This allows us to have a better quality of life with leisure time built in. This may not be true for everyone as some people still work more than one job to keep themselves financially solvent, but it is safe to say, that our lives are easier than these of our parents.

The concept of leisure in retirement is only 40 to 50 years old. As economic situations for working people improved, people started to think about how to remain active and engaged, other than by doing work.

Our days are filled not only with responsibilities, but we also have time to socialize, engage in physical activities, sports, and engage in hobbies. As mentioned before, we are better off, and, in general, better educated than the generations before us. We are also generally in better physical and mental health. But how will we pay for these golden years?

Economists tell us that although the boomers have been saving, they are not saving enough. And the cost of living has gone up quite a bit since the last generation dealt with their retirement. The traditional model of retirement was based on a combination of Social Security, pension, and some savings. Now it is mostly based on Social Security, some savings and investments. Pensions from an employer are becoming a thing of the past. We have witnessed great abuse in pension programs, which have left retirees without the promised pension at retirement.

Social Security monthly checks are the only secure part of the equation. Nine of ten seniors, who qualify to receive Social Security payments, will take them. Twenty-five percent of the recipients of monthly Social Security payments are dependent on them for 90 percent or more for their total income.

Today more than half of all workers in this country are not covered by any pension plan. And more than half of them are living from paycheck to paycheck, which means they are investing virtually nothing from that paycheck for future retirement. It is also interesting that at the time we retire and are going through so much psychological adjustment, we are leaving the careers which have been a strong part of our own self-identity. Retirement is not only a change in daily schedule; it is a change in lifestyle.

That is also the time we have to deal with our parents, if they are still alive, and their mortality, as well as our own. Many of us need to find a new direction in our lives to reflect our physical abilities, as well as our mental abilities. Our culture indoctrinates us to value ourselves and others by our productivity and the outcome of it, so if suddenly we are no longer working and producing, what are we really worth to society? It is a big adjustment psychologically for the newly retired. And compounding that are financial and physical issues.

Considering that about 70 million baby boomers will enter the "seniorhood" in the next ten years, society should plan ahead to deal with those issues. As I mentioned in previous chapters, it is a unique generation of retirees, because their expectations are higher, as is their understanding of how the government works, so they may be more demanding in their expectations.

Although times have changed, advances have been made in all areas that touch our lives, and the baby boomers hardly show any likeness to the retirees of yesteryears, we still need the same basic things. We need to feel secure, especially financially. We need to know that our health needs will be taken care of. And we need to feel respected by the society in which we live. The difference between the retirees of today and these of the generation before is that the latter hoped for the above, while the former believe it is their right to have health needs met and living standards maintained.

We live in dramatic times, in which economic structure is changing. With outsourcing, the job market is losing thousands and thousands of positions, forcing people to retire earlier than planned, or struggle in the ever-shrinking employment market seeking a position. Retirement plans need to be addressed early in our lives, so we are not caught off guard in our later years.

As a rule of thumb, you will need approximately 80 percent of your income to maintain about the same level of lifestyle. If you have written out in detail all your finances, all your projected costs, where your funds are, and how secure they are, it will be easy to follow it in the future, and you will have better control of it, and thus better able to protect it.

If we have planned to retire at the standard age of 65, and our financial investments were built and calculated with that age in mind, any unpredictable event resulting in earlier retirement, be it loss of job, illness, or any other reason, will throw off our initial calculation. So what you need to do is to factor in some of these unforeseen changes. You will need a margin of financial security, at least to cover your living expenses for perhaps, a year, without depleting your savings.

Once your financial security is in place, for your retirement, and you are fairly sure how much you will need to maintain a satisfactory standard of living, you will need to plan your future life in aspects other than just financial ones. People who do not thrive when retiring tend to be the ones who hadn't planned for their senior years, not just financially, but from a lifestyle vantage point.

So my advice is after developing a financial plan for your retirement, do the same for your social life. Write down what your hobbies are, what you enjoy doing in your free time. Are they things you would like to do in your senior years? Can you physically still do those things? You should evaluate if doing the things that you enjoy will require a great deal of money. If it requires expensive equipment, if it requires traveling, could you incorporate those expenses in your budget, even after you are retired and on fixed income?

Can you do the things that you loved doing in your middle years? Would you like to continue to play tennis or golf, for example? Can you afford those sports? Are there things you always promised yourself you would do when you retire? Do you still want to do them?

I have had clients in our agency who did not know how to occupy their time or how to fill their days with things that interested them once they retired. This can cause a sense of emptiness or depression. It is clear that the baby boomers are more involved in recreational activities, and in all likelihood will be better prepared than the generation before them, but a lesson should be learned from their predecessors.

The best situation would be to plan your residential environment to reflect your interests and hobbies. If you are living in a place where you can fulfill your needs, then find your interests in the neighborhood. Many neighborhoods are rich with programs of all sorts, such as colleges and universities, which have a full range of lectures and social programs that encourage social and intellectual interaction. YMCAs and YMHAs also have programs geared specially for the retired and elderly.

Aging couples also have to adjust to retirement, but it may be easier for them than for a single person. A couple just continues to live their life, they may decide to move to a retirement community, move out of state, away from family members, children, and grandchildren, but because they continue to be a unit, the transition is less difficult.

If major changes are made, say in living conditions, because of less income or other factors, you may need to scale down your residential situation and part with property that you loved, and you need to understand that changes are more permanent. For example, if you sell a house to move to an assisted living place, you are not likely to turn around and buy another house. That part of your life is pretty much over. It makes good sense to scale down your house to a smaller place if you are an empty nesters.

Either way you need to adapt to these changes. And if you have a partner who shares your view on the subject of making changes, it makes it that much easier to adjust.

What makes a difference in the quality of life in the senior years is the social aspect of your life. If you continue to be active socially, maintaining close contact with friends, or keeping yourself busy with recreational activities and continue to be mentally stimulated, there is a very good chance that you will maintain your mental faculties much longer than if you don't..

Many studies show that people who withdraw from social interaction, and isolate themselves from others, tend to slip into depression and do not do well health-wise. Society should provide support services to prevent elderly people from falling into situations where they get lost in the system, and become lonely, isolated, and depressed. Family members can step in and help the elderly parent or relative to find senior centers and religious centers that may provide stimulating programs and reduce isolation.

The key for successful retirement, as I said before, is to make sure that the retiree feels secure financially and physically, that he or she knows their health needs are covered, that they do not need to worry about meeting their expenses, and that they are not going to be a burden to their children and relatives.

Many western countries are providing that security for their aging population. Countries like Sweden, Canada, Denmark, Netherlands, and England provide residential care, nursing care, supplementary cost of food and medical care, as well as home care and personal aide assistance for their seniors.

Of course, none of these countries are going to face such a large increase of their aging populations and in such a short time comparable to the United States. None of those countries are going to see 70 million baby boomers joining the ranks of the seniors in the next decade. Then again, these countries are also not as rich as the United States.

The approach to the new retirement should be based on today's needs of the aging population. In previous years, we had established improved mobility settings for the disabled, such as elevators, wider doors, and ramps, buses that accommodate wheelchairs; today we ought to provide the aging population with direction of retirement planning long before they are in the position to use the different services.

While in the past we perceived the term retiree negatively, now the whole perception of a retired person needs to change. There is no question that our culture has worshipped youth for centuries. Marketing has reinforced the connection between youth and beauty. It is only in the past few decades, that the corporate world has discovered the potential profits in marketing to the overweight and the elderly. The power that 70 million consumers possess has made the corporate world take notice. And politicians should take notice as well.

Case # 20

A woman I know planned the ideal retirement for herself. She is now in her seventies, and has been retired for some time. She had a small pension, and had saved a nice nest egg for the years to come. Her investments, which she handled very conservatively, were solid. She did not take any chances with them. She also was very conservative with her monthly spending.

One of the things she enjoyed very much was traveling, so she continued to do so after retiring from her job as a buyer for a large sporting goods outfit. Through her travels in Italy, she had found a small village in Tuscany that she fell in love with, and decided to spend a few months of the year there. She rented a small house for two months, since the dollar was strong, and she ended up loving the experience. Between her monthly Social Security income, interest on her savings, and her pension, she was able maintain her apartment in the city, and live in Europe for two months a year, spending her time writing, reading, and socializing with the locals.

Every year she added another month to her stay in Italy. Currently, she is spending six months in the States, and six months in Italy. This arrangement is not depleting her savings, and brings her much joy. She wants to continue doing this as long as her health permits; and she understands that at some later point in her life she will not be able to continue this arrangement, but for now she is just having a blast. She developed wonderful friendships, and picked up gardening, which as a city girl all her life she has never done before.

This scenario may not be for everyone, but for her it was wonderful to be able to do it. The message this sends is that retirement need not to be the end of a road, empty of meaningful experiences. We can, and should, fill our days in the later years with pleasure, joy, fulfillment, and stimulating and challenging experiences.

Health Care system for the Future

Many Americans have the delusion that this country has the best health system in the world, a myth some of our politicians have been loudly promoting. It may be true that we have some of the best hospitals on the planet, especially the larger medical centers, connected with top universities, which provide the latest and most advanced treatments to those lucky ones that are fully covered by health insurance. But we are lagging behind other advanced countries in providing our citizens with good and timely health services.

Most of the other industrial nations provide universal health coverage for their citizens. The only country that does not provide health coverage is the United States even though it is the richest nation in the world. It is shameful that in this country some people are not able to go to the doctor for care they need, care that may at times save their lives. The people who have insurance coverage, for which they pay extremely high premiums, may still not be sufficiently covered for their medical needs, and the insurance companies could drop them at their whim if they develop a serious illness.

The best possible health system that we can hope for would provide medicine, preventive health care, health education, and a health system that is equally available to all Americans in their time of need. An efficient health system that will emphasize staying healthy and preventing illnesses will benefit not only our generation, but also generations to come.

The assumption that such health system is too expensive and unreachable is totally incorrect. The monies needed are already spent in the current system; what's needed is to allocate it differently and cut the profits that are currently being pocketed by large insurance companies and pharmaceutical companies.

The current system doesn't come close to covering all the people in this country. As mentioned, over 47 million Americans have no health insurance at all. Cost specialists have repeatedly said that a cover-all health system need not cost more than the current, flawed one cost.

So why is it that every time a plan is proposed for universal coverage, it is immediately shot down?

Politicians on both sides of the political spectrum are pressured by the lobbyists on behalf of the major insurance companies, the different HMOs, and other private groups that have a lot to lose if health care become nationalized. When billions of dollars are at stake, the pressure on the president and Congress is so great, that the good of the citizens becomes secondary.

What we need to do as soon as possible is the following:

1. Improve technology use, to cut waste and become more efficient.
2. Develop systems to reduce medical errors.
3. Promote healthy behavior, from infancy to ripe old age.
4. Prevent disease, not just by treating it or by curing it, but by catching it earlier.
5. Sharpen our focus on the growing problems of chronic diseases.
6. Deal with escalating cost of prescription drugs.
7. Make sure that every American has access to the health care system.

One of the first priorities is to reduce errors in the medical field. Today, there are about 195,000 deaths a year due to medical errors. It is imperative to develop and put in place systems that monitor errors, and make sure that there are guidelines and in-servicing of medical staff to decrease and eliminate medical errors. Medical errors are costly in lives, but also raise medical costs to factor in malpractice suits. And as patients, we should take care of our own health, question all that is done to us, and be educated about whatever it is that ails us.

We all read periodically about some horror story in the medical field. At time it is difficult to find accountability, especially considering the gigantic size of insurance company's bureaucracies. This has to change. The insurance companies, as well as the government agencies, and law makers, and the point of care, such as doctors, hospitals, and clinics, need to understand that they are supposed to be taking care of the patient and the consumer, and not the other way around.

This huge monstrosity called the health system is paid for by us, through taxes and through out-of-pocket co-pays. We should have a say in how it works, how it manages our health, and how much profit there should be. And I do not think it should be just a fantasy, but it needs to become reality.

If spending on health care increases three times faster than the overall economy, that so many of us are uninsured or our coverage is insufficient boggles the mind. Our elders often cannot afford medication or to visit their doctors, yet at the same time the profit-making of the insurance companies, the different HMOs, and pharmaceutical companies are skyrocketing.

As the baby boomers age, they will require and demand to be provided with preventive health services. If they should remain active, productive, and healthy, they will need those services. The only people who are supporting the current health system are the people who are benefiting financially from it. That includes insurance companies and the HMOs, as well as the politicians who benefit from financial support through the lobbyists. Elected officials, in my opinion should be held accountable by us, the voters. The time has come that the well being of the American people, young and old, should be the guiding path to decision-making regarding health needs.

Centralized Senior Centers

I worked abroad in a country that while not considered a rich nation, has a universal health system that provides coverage for every citizen from the moment they are born to the day they die.

Although I was involved in researching the morbidity and mortality rate of newborns in relation to nutrition, being exposed to the country's health system as a whole was very educational for me. It was amazing to see how a simple, uncomplicated system that is far less costly than the one we have in this country - if you want to call it a system - does not leave any of its citizens behind.

Holding a degree in gerontology and health management, I gravitated towards working with the aged after I returned to the United States. So I was shocked to see how much differently we deal with our elderly, and how fractioned our system of delivering health services to the general public, and to seniors especially, really was. While working abroad, I found that the country had many fascinating ways to deal with the needs of the elderly.

Their health system is organized to dispense health services through clinics set up throughout the cities, towns, and villages. In the cities and towns most clinics have family doctors, specialists (such as gynecologists, cardiologists, dermatologists, pediatricians, nursing services) and social workers. Smaller clinics were staffed with an internist and nursing staff, with specialists visiting weekly. Every clinic is affiliated with a hospital that is geographically close for emergency services and urgent visits to a specialist. Each hospital has many out-patient clinics specializing in every medical area.

Each clinic, no matter how small, has a pharmacy available for its members. If a member of a clinic moves to another town or city, all he or she has to do is register with the clinic near his or her new place of residence. All medical records are transferred to the new clinic, and, if need be, the new doctor can consult with the doctor who took care of the patient before.

I found that many of the elderly came into the clinic, not so much for the medical care – although that, too, was available for them when needed - but for the social interaction. They met friends there.

As a result, someone got the idea that it would be great to build senior citizen centers near the clinics. It was a great success. Elderly people socialize with their fellow seniors in the neighborhood, are served a hot lunch, and are able to use social worker services if they have a problem.

Having senior citizen centers located so close to health clinics also promotes better health practices, with visiting nurses to administer flu shots and visiting nutritionists to lecture on better eating habits and easy methods teach easy of healthy food preparation. Physical activities are taught by physical therapists that have been trained in geriatric physical needs and physical limitations.

A bond is usually formed between the elderly, and the staff of those centers, so the staff is often able to identify seniors who are in trouble, either physically or emotionally. The staff may intervene and then direct the elderly to the source that can provide them with the help they may need.

Although we have many senior citizen centers in this country, they are built and run by many different groups. Some of them are centers belonging to religious institutions, and some are run by private entities, and almost all are supplemented by government subsidies through state or federal sources.

What I would like to see in the future is the development of a unified formula that would provide the same service at all senior citizens centers. Two nutritious meals should be served daily. We could incorporate special programs, such as Alzheimer's programs, geared to stimulate the memory, or exercise programs to promote better health. For elderly people who live out of the walking distance of a senior citizen center, transportation should be provided.

Such centers should provide all services free of charge to any senior citizen that wants to take advantage of them; they should be financed by the state and federal governments. As I mentioned before, the government already finances a great deal of the programs, all we need is to centralize the different programs, and curtail some of the profits that are currently enjoyed by the administrators of such centers.

Advertising of the senior citizen centers, to make sure that all seniors in the area are aware of the availability of a center in their midst, can be done through local medical services. Information can be mailed to the elderly with their Social Security checks, providing them with a list of centers in their neighborhood.

If countries much, much poorer, are able to provide such centers for their elders, we should be able to do so too.

Good Deeds-
Sharing your wealth and goodwill with others

To the few of us who are able and willing to help others, there is no pleasure more gratifying. From many conversations that I've had with the elderly throughout the years, I always sensed the pleasure they derived from the things they gave or did, when they did not have to.

There are many ways that one can help out others. If, for example, you like reading, you can always read to others, young or old. You can share your passion, and others will appreciate that gift. Many seniors hesitate when the subject of volunteering comes up, 'What can I do for others, when I am hardly able to do things for myself?' Yet, when we continue that conversation, people do realize how much they can do to enrich other people's life.

In the nursing home one can always help, by perhaps teaching others to play chess, or checkers, or running a book club. If you like writing, you can write letters for others, who are unable to do so themselves. If you are religious, you can run the weekly prayers; you can visit bed-ridden residents, who tend to feel lonely and isolated. At times, it is easier for an elderly person to communicate with someone close to their own age, who is more likely to understand the problems they have.

If you are able and interested in volunteering in the local hospital, just by devoting one or two hours a week, your time will be well spent, and well appreciated. In the hospital one can read or tell stories to sick children or adults. Children, especially, are responsive to all you are willing to do for them. Listening to stories and playing games, will take their minds off their pain and discomfort, as well as giving their mothers or fathers a little break. In larger hospitals, well-developed volunteer departments can direct each volunteer to the most suitable area for them, and devise a personal schedule for each volunteer.

The same goes for assisted living, and residential care facilities, and retirement communities; in each of them you can find something to do for others and provide social stimulation that will give you much pleasure. You can also incorporate your hobbies and your past professional ability which can be beneficial to others.

If you are living in the community at large, there is a wide range of things for which you can volunteer. There are senior citizen centers, houses of worship, adult day care centers, local schools, public libraries, shelters, youth centers, and many other options. Community centers, where many cultural and educational programs take place on a regular basis, are another option. In churches, synagogues and mosques there are many social programs, cultural and educational programs that can always use some more volunteers, - to assist the organizers, set up for events, or help the disabled and elderly.

Visiting a lonely neighbor on a regular basis or sharing a holiday meal with someone you know, who has no family to celebrate the holiday with are great ways to help. When I worked in a nursing home, I routinely used to bring patients to my home for a Sabbath meal or holiday celebration, to include them with my family.

If you are politically oriented, there are volunteer opportunities in this area. You may volunteer in the offices of local elected officials or the offices of the affairs of the aged. You can volunteer for your candidate's campaign by making phones calls to potential voters, or to work on mailings or handing out printed materials.

You can always find ways to contribute and to help, and the satisfaction is well worth the effort. Another way to contribute is do so financially. Here too there are many options for giving. For most of us, large sums of money are not realistic when we think of donating to a cause. All the large philanthropic organizations will confirm that the bulk of the donations they receive come from small amounts of $10, $15 or $20.

If you are in a position to help others with financial giving, there are many ways to do it: through fund raising organizations (though you should do some background checking on each organization you are interested in); donating directly to a church, synagogue, local school, or senior citizen center. Check your local shelter, where people are in need of the basics, from clothing to toiletries to food.

No matter what you choose to do, do something.

The ways to give to Charity

Americans are a very generous people. A new poll by Greenwald & Associates and Synovote found that the nine out of ten families with $1 million or more have donated money or time to charitable causes. In 2006, Americans gave a record of $300 billion to causes in the United

States and around the world. No other countries came close to giving what we do. And that giving comes from all levels of income, and even the poorest among us are giving.

If and when we are blessed with financial security and our upbringing and religious beliefs emphasize the blessing of charity, then we should contribute to our communities and society at large. Many ways charitable giving to the poor, the weak, and to the needy have been established over time. If you want to give, here are some of the best ways to do it:

For those who have no blood relatives or friends to leave their estate to, there are always charities that are happy to be the recipients of your generosity. There are many charitable organizations, and it is wise to check their records before giving. Check with the Office of the Attorney General's in your state regarding the charitable organization that you are interested in; the contact information may be found at our website www.goldenyearsgolden.com Most of the information, regarding the charities can also be found on other sites on the Internet.

When you determine which charity that is closest to your heart, and you have checked that it follows the government's rules and regulations, you can put it as a beneficiary in your will or trust. You should also ask your financial advisor, if it is financially beneficial for you to continuously give smaller amounts, or to wait to leave the total amount to the charity of your choosing in your will.

You need to find out if the designated charity archives the stated goals that it presents to the potential donors. There are so many non-for-profit charitable organizations, some with very convincing marketing techniques, that even the smartest and the most business-savvy of us can fall for unrealistic pitches.

If you decide to donate, for example to an organization involved in the fight against cancer, you should first choose the specific cancer charity and then you can specify the actual venue that you would like your money to go to. For example, one may have an interest in fighting breast cancer, or funding research to eliminate leukemia, or developing techniques for early diagnosis of ovarian cancer; or funding camps for children who are battling the disease. You should specify exactly where your money should go. This will prevent your money from going into a general pot, where it will end up paying for administrative expenses, or even for office renovations and perks.

Many people save all their lives, at times denying themselves any luxuries or travel opportunities. When they know that their life is nearing the end, they just want to do the right thing and leave their money to a good cause. This is a beautiful gesture, so make sure that your money will go to the place you designate it to go.

Besides being beneficial to society and to a cause, charitable giving can also be beneficial to you. You can establish a trust for your money that pays you a monthly dividend for as long as you live, reverting to the charity that you designated once you pass away. You can find the right trust to serve you the best with the help of an estate planning lawyer. If the trust is written well, it is difficult, if not impossible, for the charity to transfer the money to anything other than to your designated projects.

If you have a home or a vacation home, or any other real estate holdings, you may want to look in into giving to charity by utilizing your real estate holdings. I recommend reading the Nov. 11, 2007 article on the subject by Vivian Marino in *The New York Times*. Many people are looking to donate their homes to charities after they are gone, if they do not have family to whom to bequeath them. In many cases, in return for their donation, they receive a monthly payment that can help them cover their living expenses, and on top of that, the charity will pay any taxes on the property.

Real estate donors can receive an income for the duration of their lives. This can be a win-win situation. To achieve this, you need to establish a charitable remainders trust. You will be receiving an income for as long as you live under such a trust, and after your passing the assets will revert to the charitable organization. There are many other benefits to charitable giving, many fairly complex, so it may be advisable to consult professionals in the field of estate planning. Mistakes in estate planning can be costly.

As with any other major decision-making that involves financial issues, your decision to bequest your money to charities should be carefully considered and legally secured. Your money should be designated to the precise beneficiary, to be used for the precise goals you have chosen. And that should be true for anything you bequest, be it real estate, trusts, or liquid money.

Second Careers and other Occupations

Many of us, especially baby boomers, are far from ready to retire and sit on the patio and just watch the sunset. Some people plan well in advance of their retirement as exactly what they will do with themselves. But for me personally, like many others, this was not an option, and we scramble to fill our retirement with many activities.

One of the options for many retirees is to starting new careers, maybe something they always wanted to do and were unable to, due to the need to provide for their families and children's education. Haven't we all entertained a dream of doing something other than what we had done throughout our professional life?

I have spoken to people who worked in different industries, some consuming long hours of the day, leaving very little time to develop hobbies and leisure activities. But after retirement, when the financial obligations have decreased and time is freed up, there are opportunities to do that which fulfills your interest, imagination, showcases your talents, and brings you joy.

A friend of mine had a dream to learn French, so after retirement, he registered for a course at the Sorbonne University, in Paris, France. He rented a studio in Paris, via the Internet, and went on to experience the most exciting three months in his life. For my friend, it was a fulfillment of a dream he had carried for a very long time. He had to start a career his early in his life to help provide for his family, which made studying in college impossible. So retirement gave him the opportunity to do the things he wanted to do, but had been unable to do until after retirement.

As I have stated earlier in this book, new retirees are still young, mentally alert, and have a great deal left to contribute to our society. There are many organizations that provide the connection between the retiree and a place of work, whether a paid job or volunteer position.

Many people await their retirement with great expectations, but when you ask them to pinpoint what is it they are planning to do when retired, their answers are very surprising. Many will say, in a much generalized way, that they will go fishing, or read all the books they did not have time to read during the time they worked. They say they will take up painting or will travel to all the places they had wanted to visit, but hadn't had time to go before. But all those great plans will fill only a fraction of the time they will have on their hands.

It is wise to preplan your retirement, activities, and interest in much the same way we preplan our retirement financially. If you would like to go back to school to study your favorite subject, it may require not only financing, but also the pinpointing of what and where will you study. Such knowledge can then be applied to a second career.

If you like history, music, art, or literature, you can take courses in those subjects; you can become an assistant to a teacher and help teach that subject to children. Again, you can do it for pay or as a volunteer. You can build a second career, without the stresses you experienced during your first one. Think of the contributions that you can make to the younger generation.

A doctor or a nurse can volunteer in long-term institutions, with consultations and educational programs, which will make use of life-long experiences and fulfill a need. This can be said about any profession of any area of knowledge. The benefit of such contributions to society is immeasurable, and the personal satisfaction is enormous.

During all the years that you have worked as an adult, your work week was most likely 40 hours or more; after you retire, regardless of whether you work for pay or as a volunteer, you can schedule your work to be much more relaxed. You can work two days or four days, you can work half days or whatever suits you. That is the beauty of a post-retirement career: you can adjust to suit your schedule and level of commitment. For seniors who are in need of additional income, to supplement their Social Security and pensions, part time work could help them with their expenses.

Look for what is FREE for Seniors

As part of reinventing retirement, look for the advantages that are available; and there are plenty of things that are free, or can be gotten for a nominal fee. The more informed you are the more advantage you can take of that. When you hear of a free service or activity, write it down and keep it. You never know when you may want to use that information.

When you read articles related to the elderly or to baby boomers, you may find useful information. Once you develop the habit of writing down useful information of possible sources for free services, programs and benefits, it will become second nature to you to retain that information, and file it in a manner in which you can easily retrieve it when you need it. I like to file bits of information and resources in files under categories such as Health Services, Entertainment, Drugs, Foods, Utilities, Sports, Supplies, etc.

A tip for special discounts: Make sure to carry a photo I.D. that gives your birthday clearly - it can be a driving license, or if you do not drive, your local Department of Motor Vehicles issues a non-driving card for identification.

Here are some things you can get for free, or for a minimal fee:

BANKS

To promote banking services, many banks offer programs that are developed with seniors in mind. For example there are CDs (Certificate of Deposits), which are accounts that provide you with a locked-in percentile for specific time. Say you want to lock in a 5-percent interest rate for six months or one year for your money, for example. If you need money to supplement your pension and Social Security for your monthly expenses, some of the CDs will pay you interest on a monthly basis, while your principle remains intact for the duration of your CD.

Ask the bank; what programs they have that will serve you best. Check if they have free checking accounts, so you will not be charged for every check you write. Most banks have direct deposit for your monthly Social Security payment. This prevents loss of checks. Many elderly have had their monthly Social Security checks stolen from their mail boxes; many of them were unable to successfully notify the Social Security offices of the loss. This made the direct deposit very desirable alternative for the elderly.

Once the direct deposit is made, and money is available to the senior, he or she can withdraw money at any time from the many ATMs everywhere. But verify if the bank charges a fee to use another bank's ATM.

In most banks, the officer of the bank will be happy to teach the elderly how to use the ATM machine, and it is advisable to maintain a relationship with representative of your bank. You can also advise your bank, that when you are not well and are unable to come to the bank, you may send someone to do it for you, with a signed note from you and a withdrawal slip authorizing that person to take out a limited amount of money.

If you are financially well-off and you need to make decisions regarding investments, every bank these days has a financial investments department, and they will be happy to send a financial adviser to talk to you in the privacy of your home. You can ask as many questions as you like, and make sure that you do not make any decisions on the spot. As with everything else, take your time.

TRANSPORTATION

Check with your Office of the Aged regarding the availability of free transportation. Many cities in the United States provide free transportation for their seniors, 65 years and older. Public transportation, such as buses, subways, and trains, charge seniors less – or don't charge seniors at all – to ride. Discounted monthly passes are usually available for seniors.

Access-a-Ride is also available for a nominal fee; in New York it costs $1.50. If you call two or three days before you need this service, in other places it may require more extended notification, then you are picked up at your home, and dropped off at your destination. The same arrangement can be made for the return trip. For Access-a-Ride you need to register initially.

You can also check with local senior citizen centers if they have organized transportation, for individual needs or organized shopping trips to malls or markets. Religious organizations also many times offer rides for elderly to activities and meals. Many churches, synagogues, and senior citizen centers receive subsidies from federal and state government to serve meals and offer recreational activities as well as transportation, free of charge.

If you have Medicaid, your doctor can arrange for you to be picked up by ambulette, or car service for appointments free of charge. In some areas, there are car pools with volunteers who will come and take seniors to doctor's appointments or shopping. This service is provided by different volunteer organization and is also free of charge. But as with all free or minimal-fee transportation available to the elderly, you have to schedule the pick-up ahead of time.

FOOD STAMPS

The federal government provides food stamps for any American in need. Food stamps are available for people who are short of funds, even if they are working. Age is not a prerequisite to qualify for food stamps. On the average, a single person can receive about $130 per month; a small percentage is entitled to over $200. Almost all supermarkets accept food stamps, and many smaller grocery stores are currently accepting food stamps as well.

When applying for food stamps, you need to prove place of residence, and be able to show your income and expenses. It usually takes a month for the documentation to be processed. But if there is an emergency, food stamps can be gotten in few days. One can only buy food with food stamps. You may not purchase detergents, toiletries, paper goods, such as paper towels, toilet paper, napkins, etc.; cigarettes and medical supplies cannot be purchased by food stamps, either.

Many elderly living on a fixed income, often on just their Social Security entitlement, find that food stamps are very helpful. Food stamps can be received as per need, indefinitely or to help someone through a rough time.

Check in the General Sources of Information at the end of this book where and how to apply for food stamps. You can see more information on our website www.goldenyearsgolden.com .

MEALS ON WHEELS

Meals on Wheels is one of the better known services that delivers fresh, ready-to-eat meals to the elderly in their own homes. The meals are well balanced and nutritious. Many times the food brought to the elderly on a daily basis is not only a source of good nutrition, but a source of social interaction. At times, seeing the volunteer may be the only human contact they have all day.

Meals on Wheels is not the only agency providing ready-to-eat meals to the elderly; there other agencies providing similar services.

If you need to find out what organizations deliver meals to homes in your neighborhood, you can get the information from your state and city government Office for the Aged. Some of the meals delivered may have a nominal fee, no more than a dollar or two. The meals include a hot main dish, salad, bread, a fruit, and a pint of milk.

Most meals that are delivered to the elderly are prepared with the supervision of a nutritionist, with general health needs taken into account, such as low-sodium, and reduced-sugar foods. If you have nutritional restrictions, make sure to ask the provider of this service if their food is appropriate for your needs.

HOT MEALS

Hot meals are also available at senior citizen centers, religious centers, and at other facilities. There are places whose sole reason of existence is to provide meals for those who need them. These places serve the population in need, and age is not a factor here. Any one in need of a meal can come in, and eat a hot, nutritious meal. To find such a center, contact your mayor's office, the Office of the Aged, or the social services department in the hospital closest to you. Some of these centers require a nominal fee for the meal, which is served in a social environment, and promotes social interaction between the participants. Thus, it serves two purposes: it provides a hot and nutritious meal, and provides a friendly social environment for the participants, who at times do not have any other social interaction.

Many religious centers provide hot meals daily to elderly people, and to members of their churches or synagogues who are in need. It is mostly open to anyone needing a hot meal. Many religious centers, churches, synagogues, and mosques run a free kitchen during holidays, and tend to have holiday celebrations that are open to all who wish to take part in them.

CULTURAL EVENTS AND MUSEUMS

In every city and town in this country there are hundreds of cultural events taking place on any given day. And you too can enjoy them, many times free of charge, or for a minimal charge. Many theaters are subsidized by the government, with a stipulation that they provide a fixed number of tickets for the elderly.

Some senior citizen centers receive tickets to some cultural events to give away to the seniors. The events may include theater shows, concerts, lectures, exhibits, etc. Find out the nearest senior citizen center in your area, so you can take advantage of these free events.

Universities in your city or town are also a good source of cultural events that are free of charge. Put yourself on their mailing list for future events. Most of the universities and colleges are very welcoming to seniors and will invite them to take advantage of their entertainment events. In many universities the seniors can audit courses of interest free of charge. That, at times, is a fulfillment of a dream to a senior who may have worked all his life and never had an opportunity to take advantage of higher education. This may be challenging, stimulating, and very enriching. And in most cases, free.

Follow the local newspapers for events happening around town. There are theater performances, concerts, art galleries, and exhibits in the local museums. Call any of these places and ask if they offer free admission to senior citizens. Movie theaters offer discount tickets almost uniformly, but at times they will offer, maybe matinee at half price, or a fraction of the actual cost of the ticket, on a specific day.

Many restaurants that have a day or two a week during which they serve lunches or dinners at half a price for seniors; some will have a standing price discount for seniors. Others offer an early-bird discount to seniors. Great deals of restaurants have a senior section on their menu, with reduced prices, at times with reduced-size meals.

Museums throughout the country have reduced tickets costs for seniors. Many museums have a policy that people aged 65 years and over can enter free of charge. Call each museum individually and check with them as to their policy regarding seniors.

Some cities, New York City for example, have special weekly or monthly passes for seniors, at a reduced price, allowing, you to visit several museums.

Sports events too, may provide for free or reduced tickets for the seniors. Local baseball, basketball, and hockey teams also may have events that can be enjoyed by the elderly. Some have an early game once a week with special reduced prices for seniors.

Music schools, conservatories, and ballet schools all have open performances that the audience, regardless of age, is encouraged to attend. I have attended many performances at the world famous Juilliard, in New York City, free of charge, and it is wonderful to see budding talent that will eventually become top performers in their field. Philharmonic orchestras, will almost always have their rehearsals before an audience, at a fraction of the cost, or free for seniors.

If you have a lot of friends, or if you reside in a nursing home, residential care, or assisted living facility, you can establish a group which allows you to ask for special rates. Small theaters that are supported by grants and subsidies are obligated to provide a specified percentage of their tickets to seniors, and schools, free of charge.

Libraries also may be a source of cultural events that are free of charge. Many times public libraries will host film presentations, lectures, readings by authors or professors from local schools.

Local zoo, botanical gardens, visiting circuses, opera house, concert halls, and local symphonies, if your city has them, all will have special rates or free tickets for the elderly. National parks also offer special deals for seniors, so before you take a trip, check what benefits you are eligible for.

To learn more, call or visit the venues of the shows and programs and ask if there are specials for seniors, and how you can obtain a free, or reduced ticket. Most of the above discounts and free-of-charge entry to events are available to every person aged 65 years and older regardless of financial status.

RENT INCREASE EXEMPTION

If you or your parent are over 65 years old and of limited income, you are entitled in some states to apply for an exemption of rent increases, if you are approved, your rent will not be increased from the time of your approval. You can check through the Department for the Aging in your state for the Senior Citizen Rent Increase Exemption

Program (SCRI). In your state, the program may be under a different name, but the benefit to you is the same.

You have to be recertified each year to qualify for continuation of this benefit. You have to keep on top of the schedule, and a month before your certification for rent freeze lapses, you should reapply for recertification. Some of the SCRI offices will send you a reminder, and a list of requested information and documentation that it is required of you to recertify your exemption. The final responsibility for timely recertification is yours. So always mark your calendar, eleven months ahead, to call the agency. Considering that rent increases are on the average of 3 to 5 percent per year, this can be a significant savings for you. For more information go to the Office of the Aging in your state.

Chapter 11 -
Last Word

How would you summarize this book? How do you tie the information together to become a road map to guide you, or someone you love, to an easier, better, and more informed-decision making, such as developing a plan for the later years of your life? How do we help you to plan ahead so you can live with the maximum amount of independence and the least amount of stress?

To begin with, you should know what services and programs are out there, in your community at large, which can help you in your particular situation. This book touches on many of those options. And what is important for you to know is that you are not alone, millions of people are grappling with the same issues as you.

We are actually at a turning point in our society, at the doorstep of new developments that will translate into huge changes in our everyday lives. To begin with, we, the seniors who are 55 and over, are becoming a larger percentage of the 300 millions of the United States. From now on, any elected government, be it Democratic or Republican, will have to make decisions that reflect the needs, not only of the general public, but specifically the elderly.

It is the right of every American, young and old to be able to live safely, with free education for every child; every person should have health coverage, decent housing, and should not go hungry in the richest country in the world.

We have moved away from the lifestyle our grandparents and their grandparents practiced. While doing that, we have lost the direct connection of taking responsibilities for one another. This does not mean that we should stop advancement and modernization, but we shouldn't lose sight of the connection we have to others.

In previous generations, there was a closely-knit family - grandmothers always lived with members of their immediate family, and their care was secured by her loved ones. It is a totally different world now; most people communicate and keep in touch through electronic devices. In many cases, after a telephone call or an email, the senior goes back to a lonely daily life without true human contact. America should provide the elderly with a better reality. And being that we are Americas we all hold responsibility to care for our elders, directly or indirectly.

We should use the same notion that Senator Hillary Clinton put forward in her book "It Takes a Village". Although she speaks about raising children, and how the whole village takes responsibility for the welfare of every child, we should apply the same formula to seniors. We should all be responsible for the elderly, and no senior living alone, should be truly alone. When I say all of us, I mean not only me and you; I include the doctor and nurse, who provide the care for that senior. I mean the next-door neighbor, the mailman, and the people running the local senior citizen center. The clergy should reach out to the lonely, and encourage them to join the local community and decrease their isolation.

While waiting for societal changes to take root and build a much-needed structure in the caring and providing for the wellbeing of our elders, we should familiarize ourselves with what is available now, and what can immediately improve the quality of life of your parent, your aging relative, or yourself. You can pick and choose all you think can be helpful in your specific situation from this book. And I do hope that it will be a great deal of help.

I have presented the reader with the different options for residential situations, and I hope that my assessments of pros and cons were of benefit to you at the time you are debating the choices. But as with making any important choice in any area of your life, take your time in evaluating each option, compare, and consider your specific physical, financial, familial, social and religious situations. Only after taking the time to check and recheck, can you make the right decision.

I hope that while reading this book, you will come away with the sense of how much the retirement notions have changed, from the retirement that our parents experienced, when they actually were able to retire. Today's retiree is a new breed. An average retiree is much more engaged physically and socially, as well as intellectually. In general, the retiree continues to be active, in many cases continuing to work, if not full time, then part time. He or she is likely to have hobbies and exercise on a regular basis.

America is slowly evolving to recognize the contribution that seniors make to the society around them. Many retirees volunteer, helping other seniors, as well as the society at large. They volunteer in schools and hospitals, and are rich in knowledge and abilities that move the economy. It is beneficial for all us to benefit from this wealth of knowledge and contributions. It should not be wasted.

The idea of the book is to help you to find the information that you need to help you or your loved one. To make it easier for you to find specific information you need for your state, I developed a list of contacts and resources, divided by state, with information grouped into general easy-to-find categories, which can be located at the end of this book and on our website www.goldenyearsgolden.com .

I hope this book will serve you well, for many years. Although some of the material will require updates, such as eligibility thresholds, deductions, and raises in fees and costs, most of the information will be applicable for many years.

I devoted my life to working with the elderly, and through the years, the seniors that I was privileged to meet have enriched my life, and taught me a great deal. My philosophy, which I preached to my staff, when working with the elderly was, and still is, love the elderly, respect them, help them, be kind to them, and treat them well, because one day we will be in their shoes and will like the same treatment bestowed upon us. Twenty years later, I will still preach the same philosophy.

When researching and writing this book, I realized how lucky I have been to work with people who enriched my life, as I hope, I did theirs. It is not in every profession that you can do right for another human being, and know that they appreciate what you do for them. And it is not in every profession that what you do for another human being makes a direct difference in another person's life.

If there is one thing that I would like you to come away with after reading this book, I would like it to be the fact that our society, although very complex and far from perfect, still offers seniors opportunities for a very rich life. The key is to make your life, or the life of your parent, as rich as it can possibly be. When we are fortunate to have a loving family surrounding us, it makes our life much easier in our later years. But the seniors who are alone also can have a meaningful life, if they are embraced by the community. I do believe that we all can make our "golden years golden."

THINGS YOU SHOULD KNOW:

For your benefit, I am providing you with a list of specialists, which you may need in your later years, as well as description of services they provide:

ALERGIST / IMMUNOLOGIST: (Disorder of the immune system) Services provided: Allergy testing, treatment of allergies, asthma or other related disorders.

ANESTHESIOLOGIST: (Pain control) Services provided: Sedation before surgery or a procedure, non-surgical pain management.

CARDIOLOGIST: (Heart and blood vessel disorders) Services provided: Treatment of coronary artery disease, high blood pressure, heart failure, or other heart or circulatory problems.

DERMATOLOGIST: (Disorders of the skin, hair and nails) Services provided: Evaluation and treatment of a rash, skin changes, moles and skin cancer, cosmetic procedures.

EMERGENCY MEDICINE PHYSICIAN: (Trauma, emergency care) Services provided: Emergency services related to an accident, poisoning, heart attack, stroke or other serious medical condition.

ENDOCRINOLOGIST: (Hormone disorders) Services provided: Treatment of diabetes, obesity, thyroid disease and related disorders.

GASTROENTEROLOGIST: (Disorders of the digestive system and liver) Services provided: Treatment of heartburn, diarrhea and constipation, inflammatory bowl disease, and other gastrointestinal disorders.

GENETICIST: (Inherited disorders) Services provided: Genetic testing and counseling.

GERIATRICIAN: (Aging process) Services provided: Treatment of a number of age related diseases, including Alzheimer's disease.

HEMATOLOGIST: (Blood disorders) Services provided: Treatment of anemia, leukemia, lymphoma, bleeding or clotting disorders.

INFECTIOUS DISEASE SPECIALIST: (Viral, bacterial and other infectious diseases) Services provided: Treatment of infectious diseases, including HIV or AIDS, or an infection not responding to therapy, unexplained illness after travel.

NEPHROLOGIST: (Kidney disorders, high blood pressure) Services provided: Treatment of kidney failure, kidney stones or other kidney disorders, and high blood pressure.

NEUROLOGIST: (Disorders of the brain and nervous system) Services provided: Treatment of stroke, Parkinson's disease, Alzheimer's disease, multiple sclerosis or other nervous system disorders.

OBSTETRICIAN / GYNECOLOGIST: (Women's health) Services provided: Treatment of menopause symptoms, sexual dysfunction and female reproductive disorders.

ONCOLOGIST: (Non surgical treatment of cancer) Services provided: Treatment of cancer, some oncologists specialize by cancer type.

OPHTHALMOLOGIST: (Care of the eyes) Services provided: Vision correction and treatment of cataracts, glaucoma, and age related macular degeneration and other vision disorders.

ORTHOPEDIST: (Musculoskeletal and joint disorders) Services provided: Surgical treatment of bones and joints, such as fracture repair and joint replacement.

OTOLARYNGOLOGIST / EAR, NOSE, THROAT (ENT): (Disorders of the ears, nose and throat and neck) Services provided: Treatment of hearing loss, ringing in the ears, vertigo, sinusitis, throat cancer, and some head and neck disorders.

PHYSIATRIST: (Rehabilitation and treatment of physical disabilities and musculoskeletal disorders)

Services provided: Rehabilitation after injury or illness, such as heart attack, fracture or brain injury, and treatment of musculoskeletal pain.

PSYCHIATRIST / PSYCHOLOGIST: (Mental, addictive and emotional disorders) Services provided: Treatment of anxiety, depression, dementia and addiction and other mental illnesses.

PULMONOLOGIST: (Lung disorders) Services provided: Treatment of lung disorders, including chronic obstructive pulmonary disease (COPD) and lung cancer.

RADIOLOGIST: (Imaging to diagnose disease, interventional procedures) Services provided: Application and interpretation of tests such as X-rays, ultrasound, magnetic resonance imaging (MRI) or computerized tomography (CT).

RHEUMATOLOGIST: (Immune diseases of joints, muscles and bones) Services provided: Treatment of arthritis, connective tissue diseases, vasculitis, or other related diseases.

SURGEON: (Surgical treatment of diseases and disorders) Services provided; surgical diagnosis and treatment, some surgeons specialize by condition or organ, such as plastic surgeons or cardiovascular surgeons.

UROLOGIST:(Disorders of the urinary and urogenital tracts) Services provided: Treatment of bladder, kidney and prostate conditions and other urinary tract disorders.

The above list was compiled by the Mayo Clinic Women's Health Source, publishes July 2007.

Among other things that you should be able to have at your fingertips is you local senior citizens centers, the closest hospital, and phone numbers of the Agency of Aging local office. All relevant numbers should be kept ready available, preferable displayed in a visible place, such as on the refrigerator. Periodic review of the numbers should be made, and any numbers that are not relevant should be discarded, and new relevant numbers added.

RESOURCES

NATIONAL GOVERNMENT OFFICES and AGENCIES

Relating to the Elderly and Seniors

Eldercare Locator   800-677-1116
www.eldercare.gov

The Elder Locator is a free national directory assistance public service that helps you to locate different aging services in every community throughout the United States. Among the services you can find information about are: Alzheimer's, different Hot Lines, transportation information, if you have any housing option question, such as subsidized housing availability of different options. Information regarding home health services, and different providers, can also be gotten from Eldercare Locator..

USA.gov for Seniors
www.seniors.gov
Washington, D.C.

Fifty-Plus lifelong Fitness
P.O. Box 20230 Stanford,CA94309
605-323-6160
www.50plus.org

National Center for Assisted Living
Washington, D.C
202-842-4444
www.alfa.org

National Institute on Aging
Bethesda, MD
888-222-2225
www.nia.nih.gov

National Hospice and Palliative Care Organization
Alexandria, Va.
703-837-1500
www.nhpco.org

AARP
601 E. Street NW
Washington, DC 20049
Toll Free: 1-888-687-2277
Web site: www.aarp.org
Advocacy organization for people 50 years and older.

Administration on Aging
www.aoa.gov

Area Agency on Aging
www.n4a.org
1-800-677-1116

ALZHEIMER'S ADDICIATION
225 North Michigan Avenue, Suite 1700
Chicago, IL 60601-7633
Toll Free: 1-800-272-3900
Web site: www.alz.org
The site provides information on research and support site.

ALZHEIMER'S DISEASE EDUCATION AND REFERRAL
CENTER
P.O. Box 8250
Silver Springs, MD 20907-8250
Telephone: 1-800-438-4380
Web site: www.alzheimers.org
Organization that provides information to families, and to professionals.

Family Caregiver Alliance
www.caregiver.org

FAMILY 4 CARE
Web site: www.families4care.org
Family Alliance for Compassionate Eldercare.

NATIONAL ACADEMY OF ELDER LAW
1604 North Country Club Rd.
Tucson, AZ 85716
Telephone: 1-520-881-4005
Web site: www.naeia.org
Organization helping you to find attorneys specializing in legal issues relating to the elderly.

NATIONAL COUNCIL ON THE AGING
300 D. Street, SW, Suite 801
Washington, D.C. 20024
Telephone: 1-202-479-1200
Web site: www.ncoa.org
Organization promoting self-determination and health of the elderly.

NATIONAL LONG-TERM CARE OMBUDSMAN RESOURCE CENTER
1424 16th Street, NW, Suite 202
Washington, DC 20036
Telephone: 1-202-332-2275
Web site: www.ltcombudsman.org
Site provides the listing of all states ombudsman's offices.

Medicare Rights
www.medicarerights.gov

HOSPICE CARE
National Hospice and Palliative Care Organization
www.nhpco.org

HOSPICE CARE
American Hospice Foundation
2120 L Street, NW, Suite 200
Washington, DC 20037
Web site: www.americanhospice.org
Hospice information organization, providing advocacy and educational
information related to hospice care.

HOSPICE CARE
National Hospice and Palliative Care Organization
1700 Diagonal Road, Suite 625
Alexandria, VA 22314
Telephone: 1-703-837-1500
Web site: www.nho.org
Organization promoting quality end-of-life care.

NURSING HOMES
www.medicare.gov/nhccompare.gov

MEDICARE
1-800-MEDICARE
1-800-633-4227

SOCIAL SECURITY
1-800-772-1213

DEPARTMENT of Health and Human Services
Office of the Inspector General
1-800-447-8477
Office for Civil Rights
1-800-368-1019

DEPARTMENT of VETERANS AFFAIRS
1-800-827-1000

LONG TERM CARE
American Association of Homes and Services for the Aging
2519 Connecticut Avenue, NW
Washington, DC 20008
Telephone: 1-202-783-2242
Web site: www2.aahsa.org
Association for the advancement, of quality affordable care for seniors.

LONG TERM CARE
American Health Care Association
1201 L. Street, N.W.
Washington, DC 20005
Telephone: 1-202-842-4444
Web site: www.ahca.org
Association representing long term care providers.

LONG TERM CARE LIVING
www.longtermcareliving.com
Source of consumer information about long term care.

MEMBER OF THE FAMILY
Web site: www.memberofthefamily.net
National Nursing Home Watch List.
Information about Medicare and Medicaid certified nursing homes.

NATIONAL ASSOCIATION OF PROFESSIONAL GERIATRIC CARE MANAGERS
1604 N. Country Club Road
Tucson, AZ 85716-3102
Telephone: 1-520-881-8009
Web site: www.caremanager.org
Association of professionals specializing in assisting families with long term care planning.

NATIONAL CENTER FOR ASSISTED LIVING
1201 L Street, N.W.
Washington, DC 20005
Telephone: 1-202-842-4444
Web site: www.ncal.org
Provides consumer information regarding assisted living.

NATIONAL CITIZENS COALITION FOR NURSING HOME REFORM
Web site: www.nccnhr.org
Advocacy organization to promote quality in long term care.

ELDER ABUSE
Clearinghouse on Abuse and Neglect of the Elderly (CANE)
National Center on Elder Abuse
1201 15th Street, NW, Suite 350
Washington, DC 20005-2842
Telephone: 1-202-898-2586
Web site: www.elderabusecenter.org
Information and assistance on issues related to abuse of seniors. Web site provides information to elder abuse on.

MENTAL HELP SOURCES

National Institute of Mental Health
1-866-615-6464
www.nimh.nih.gov

National Foundation for Depressive Illness
800-248-1265
www.depression.org

National Alliance for the Mentally Ill
800-950-6264
www.nami.org

Depression and Bipolar Support Alliance
800-826-3632
www.dbsalliance.org

American Association for Geriatric Psychiatry
301-654-7850
www.aagponline.org

National Mental Health Association
This organization addresses all aspects of mental health and mental illness. The NMHA is working to improve the mental health of all Americans, through advocacy, education, research and service.
www.nmha.org

National Alliance on Mental Illness
This is the nation's largest organization dedicated to improving the lives of persons living with serious mental illness and their families. NAMI was founded in 1979 and since became the nation's voice on mental illness.
The organization mission is through advocacy, research, support and education, promote better mental health.
www.nami.org

National Institute of Health
NIH was founded in 1887, and it is today one of the world's foremost medical research centers, as well as Federal focal point for medical research in the United States. The NIH comprises 27 separate institutes and centers, and is one of eight health agencies of the Public Health Services. The goal of NIH is to acquire new knowledge to help prevent, detect, diagnose, and treat disease and disability, from the simple cold to the rarest genetic disorder.
www.nimg.nih.gov

National Schizophrenia Foundation
NSF is a not for profit consumer based education and support agency. It focuses on public awareness, information and peer support.
www.NSFoundation.org

Anxiety Disorders Association of America
This organization promotes the prevention, treatment and cure of anxiety disorders, and to improve the lives of people suffering from them.
www.adaa.org

**American Association of Homes
and Services for the Aging**
2519 Connecticut Avenue
N.W., Washington, D.C. 20008
Telephone: 1-202-783-2242
Fax: 1-202-783-2255

Victims of Fraud and Scam's
Public Disclosure Program
1800-289-9999

National Fraud Hotline
1-800-876-7060

Federal Trade Commission
1-877-382-4357

Aging with Dignity

This organization publishes "Five Wishes", which is an easy to use legal document that helps adults of all ages to plan for the care they want in case they become seriously ill.
www.agingwithdignity.org

Caring Connection

This organization is a program of the National Hospice and Palliative Care. It is geared to improve care at the end of life, and it is supported by a grant from The Robert Wood Johnson Foundation. Caring Connection provides a variety of free resources on end of life issues.
www.caringinfo.org

Hospice Foundation of America

This foundation provides help to those who cope personally or professionally with terminal illness, death, and the process of grief and bereavement.
www.hospicefoundation.org

Department of Veterans Affairs
National Center for Post-Traumatic Stress Disorder

This organization was created to advance the clinical care and social welfare of American's veterans through research, education, and training in the science, diagnosis, and treatment of PTSD, and stress related disorders.
www.ncptsd.va.gov

National Institutes of Health Medline Plus

This organization is a resource of health information from the world's largest medical library. Health professionals and consumers alike can depend on it for information that is authoritative and up to date. Medline Plus receives his extensive information from National Institutes of Health and other sources on over 700 diseases and conditions. On the site of Medline Plus you can find a list of hospitals, physicians, and a medical dictionary, health information in Spanish, extensive information on prescription and nonprescription drugs, health information from the media, and links to thousands of clinical trials.
http://www.nlm.nih.gov/medlineplus/stress.html

Destination RX

If you not sure what is the generic equivalent to your medication, you can check on this site by typing in your brand medication, you will get the information about your drug, the cost, and any side effects warnings, that may occur by using this medication. It will also give you all the generic options that are on the market, equivalent to your brand drug.

www.drx.com

Consumers Reports Best Buy Drugs

On this site you are able to find overviews of how medication work, and interact. You can see the prices of medications, and their generic equivalent. Also on this site you can find illnesses, and the different drugs being used to treat them. The drugs are compared to alternatives by their component and price.

www.crbestbuydrugs.org

GLOSSARY

WORDS DEFINITIONS

ACTIVITIES OF DAILY LIVING (ADL): A benchmark to measure a persons ability to care for him or herself, dressing, bathing, preparing and eating, with out assistance.

ASSISTANT LIVING: A facility providing living accommodations, such as room and board, can be and apartment, where you live independently. The services provided in Assistant Living vary from one facility to another, but most will provide recreational facility, transportation, laundry services, etc.

ADULT DAY CARE: Daily care provided in non residential situations. The care can be provided either to provide special care programs, such as programs for Alzheimer's patients, or custodial programs to provide respite to the main care giver.

ADVANCE MEDICAL DIRECTIVE: A document directing your medical care, in the event that you are not able to make the decisions, or instruct the medical staff regarding your care.

ALZHEIMER'S DISEASE: It is a degenerative disease of the brain, that manifests itself by loss of cognitive functions.

ANCILLARY SERVICES: Additional services that are provided in nursing homes, assisted living facilities, above the basic custodial care provided in all such facilities. Among such additional services, the facility may provide skilled nursing services, rehabilitative services, hospice programs, or other services.

CERTIFIED NURSES AIDE: A trained professional that has been certified to work with patients, although, is not a licensed nurse.

CONTINUING CARE RETIREMENT COMMUNITY: A facility or a community that presents an residential option to the senior providing multi- level living situations. It may provide full range of choices, such as independent living options as well as, skilled nursing, assistant living, special units dealing with specific needs, such as Alzheimer's patients, etc.

CUSTODIAL CARE: Care provided by a none-skilled personal, such as activities of daily living, bathing, food preparation, and feeding, helping with household choirs, ambulation, etc.

DEDUCTIBLE: The amount you or your parent must pay for health care and prescription.

DO NOT RESUSITATE (DNR): A document that provides advance directive to your doctors in the hospital, or other skilled care facility, that you do not wish to have cardiopulmonary resuscitation be administered, in case of suffering sudden cardiac arrest, or respiratory arrest.

DURABLE MEDICAL EQUIPMENT: Medical equipment that may be ordered by your doctor, for your use at home. Such equipment may be a walker, wheelchairs, or hospital bed, etc.

ELIMINATION PERIOD: It represents the period of time that the patient pays out of packet in long term facility, before his or hers insurance kicks in.

FORMULARY: A list of drugs covered by your plan.

GERIATRIC CARE MANAGER: A trained professional that assists in long term care planning, and seeks out the most suitable facility for the elderly that hired him, or her.

GUARDIANSHIP: An appointee by the court that will represent, and manage the affairs of an elderly person, that has been deemed incompetent.

HEALTH CARE PROXY: A document that is a advance directive that assigns a person to be the representative of yours, in making medical and health care decisions on your behalf, in case you are not able to make those decisions.

HOME EQUITY CONVERSION MORTGAGE PROGRAM (HECM): A reversed mortgage program federally insured (make sure to check that out, regarding the financial company you dealing with). In this program the senior, who needs to be 62 years, and over, receives a loan for long term care, based on the equity of his or hers home.

HOME HEALTH AIDE: A person trained to provide home care to a person that need help with activities of daily living, such as bathing, dressing, food preparation, shopping, cleaning, accompany patient to doctors appointment..

HOSPICE: A facility or program that provides care for the terminally ill. The program provides care focusing on pain, an emotional support to the patient and family.

INDEPENDENT LIVING COMMUNITY: A community that consists of independent residential units, at times sharing recreational facilities, and the residents have to be 55 years and older.

INPATIENT REHABILITATION FACILITY: Hospital or Nursing Home that provide an intensive rehabilitation program.

INSTITUTION: A facility that provides long term care, such as a nursing facility or skilled nursing facility.

LIVING WILL: A document instructing that no extraordinary life prolonging measures will be taken on the behalf of the person making the that directive, in the event that she or he become incapacitated, and unable to make their wishes known.

LONG TERM CARE: Services that help people with or personal needs, and activities of daily living, for prolong time. This type of care can be provided either in the person home, in the community, or in different facilities, including nursing homes, and assisted living facilities. Most long term care is custodial care.

LONG TERM CARE FACILITY: A residential option for the elderly that are not able to remain in their home, and are required assistance for their personal care, also called assistance in activities of daily living, as well in nursing care.

LONG TERM CARE INSURANCE: An insurance policy providing coverage for long term care, which can be provided in the policy holder's home, or in a long term facility, such as assistant living, skilled nursing facility, or a nursing home.

LOOK BACK PERIOD: The period of three to five years prior to applying for Medicaid. Money transferred during that period, will trigger the applicant, and make him or her Medicaid ineligible.

MEDICAID: Medicaid is a joint federal and state program that helps with medical and health needs of people with limited income and resources. This program may vary from state to state, but most health care expenses will be covered, if you qualify.

MEDICARE: Federally funded health insurance, that is provided to people 65 years and older. Disabled people younger then 65 years, also may qualify.

MEDICARE ADVANTAGE PLAN (Part C): A Medicare plan offered by a private insurance company that is contracted with Medicare to provide both Medicare Part A and B.

MEDICARE COST PLAN: In this plan one can get services outside the plan's network. Medicare covered services will be paid for by Medicare, as if under the original plan.

MEDICARE HEALTH MAINTENANCE ORGANIZATION (HMO) Similar to Medicare Advantage Plan Part C, available in some areas of the country. The HMO must cover both Part A and Part B health care. In most HMO's plans you may only use the doctors, specialists, or hospitals from their plan lists, except in emergency situations. There is a possibility that your costs may be lower than in the original Medicare plan.

MEDICARE PRESCIPTION DRUG PLAN (PART D): This plan stands on its own, and adds prescription drug coverage to the original Medicare Plan. Those plans can be provided by private insurance companies, or through health services providing companies, that are approved by Medicare.

MADIGAP PALICY: Medicare supplement insurance, sold by private insurance companies to fill a gap between the Medicare coverage and the cost of health services.

NURSING HOME: Long term care facility, can be skilled care facility, and have many special programs.

OMBUDSMAN: An advocate on behalf of the elderly, in the facility, nursing or assistant living. The ombudsman will advocate for the resident in disputes against the facility, and may investigate residents complain, or abuse.

PENALTY PERIOD: The time period, in which the Medicaid applicant is ineligible for enrollment, due to transfer of the applicant's property for less then fair market value.

POINT-of-SERVICES: A Health Maintenance Organization (HMO) option that lets you use doctors and hospitals outside your plan for additional cost.

PREVENTIVE SERVICES: Health care to prevent illness, or detect illness in its early stages, when treatment is most effective.

PRIMARY CARE DOCTOR: Primary care doctor is the doctor to provide you general health care, keep you healthy, and if needed, direct you to a specialist if special care is needed.

PROGRAMS OF ALL-INCLUSIVE CARE FOR THE ELDERLY (PACE): This program combines medical, social, and long term care services to help frail and ill elderly, to stay independently, and live in their home and community for as long as it is possible. All that while receiving high quality of care. PACE is available only in states that have chosen to provide this plan under Medicaid.

QUALIFYING HOSPITAL STAY: The patient's hospital stay, occurring prior to patient's admission to a nursing home, as required by Medicare, before it will pay for nursing home care. To qualify the patient has to be hospitalized at least three days, consecutive.

REFERRAL: A written order by your primary care doctor for you to see a specialist, or special services. In many HMO's you need to get a referral before you can get care from anybody, other then your primary care doctor. If you do not get a referral prior to receiving the health service, you may be liable for the cost.

RESIDENT ASSESSMENT INSTRUMENT: A form that used to evaluate a resident in a long term facility on his or hers physical and emotional abilities.

RESIDENTIAL CARE FACILITY: A facility that provides room and board, and very limited other services. It may have a nurse visiting to distribute medication, transportation may be provided for doctors visits and shopping. No skilled services are provided in residential care facility.

291

RESIDENT'S REPRESENTATIVE: A person representing a resident in dealing with the facility. In most cases it is a family member or the resident or a friend.

RESPITE CARE: Care provided to a patient for short period of time, to give respite to the permanent care giver.Some facilities have a special program providing respite care.

REGISTEREDS NURSE: A highly trained and skilled nursing professional that is licensed by the state in which she practicing nursing care.

RETIREMENT COMMUNITY: A community of independent living, sharing recreational facilities, and to be a resident in such community, one has to be 55 years and older.

SKILLED NURSING FACILITY CARE (SNF): This a facility that provides care that requires daily involvement of skilled nursing and rehabilitation personnel. In such facility the patient is able to receive services such as, intravenous services, physical therapy, occupational therapy, assistance with activities of daily living, such as bathing, dressing and feeding.

SUPPLENTAL SECURITY INCOME (SSI): A monthly benefit paid by Social Security to people with limited income and resources who are disabled, blind or age 65 and older. SSI benefits are not the same as Social Security benefits.

BIBLIOGRAPHY

POSITIVE AGING by Robert Hill, 2005

OPTIMAL/ SUUCCESSFUL AGING by Hill Wahlim, 1995

IMPAIRED or DEFICIT AGING by Peterson, 1999

DISEASED OF AGING by Hans Kugler, Earl R. Mindell , 1984

CARING FOR YOUR PARENTS: The Complete AARP Guide by Hugh Delehanty and Eleanor Ginzler, 2005

THE ELDERCARE HANDBOOK: DIFFICULT CHOICES, COMPASSIONATE SOLUTIONS by Stella Mora Henry RN, 2006

ELDERCARE for DUMMIES by Rachelle Zuckerman, PhD, 2003

WHAT DO YOU DO WHEN YOUR PARENTS LIVE FOREVER
By Dan and Lavinia Cohn-Sherbok, 2007

ELDER RAGE by Jacqueline Marcell, 2001

ELDERCARE 911 : The Caregivers Complete Handbook for Making Decisions By Susan Berman and Judith Rappaport-Musson, 2008

WHEN SOMEONE YOU LOVE NEEDS NURSING HOME, ASSISTED LIVING, OR IN-HOME CARE by Robert F. Bornstein, PhD and Mary A. Languirand, PhD. 2002

WHY SURVIVE? Being Old in America by Robert N. Butler, MD. 1975, 2002

THE MERCK MANNUAL OF HEALTH and AGING, by Beers, Mark H. and Thomas V. Jones, 2004

MEDICAID PLANNING HANDBOOK: A Guide to Protecting Your Family Assets from Catastrophic Nursing Home Cost by Alexander A. Bove, Jr., 1996

HOW TO CARE FOR AGING PARENTS by Virginia Morris, 2004

CARING FOR YOURSELF WHILE CARING FOR YOUR AGING PARENTS By Clair Berman, 2005

CARE GIVERS SURVIVAL MANUAL: How to Care for Your Aging Parents without Losing Yourself by Alexis Abramson, 2004

CAREGIVING: A Step by Step Resources for Caring the Cancer Patient at Home by Peter Honts and Julia A. Boncher, American Cancer Society Staff and Volunteers, American Cancer Society, 2000

DOING THE RIGHT THING: Taking Care of Your Elderly Parents, Even if They Didn't Take Care of You by Roberta, Penguin 2005

NEWSLETTER: Care-Givers Home Companion Pederson Publishing, P.O. Box 693 Southport, CT 06890-0693 Advice and Tips, online www.caregivershome.com

PROTECTING AMERICA'S HEALTH: The FDA Business and One Hundred Years of Regulation by Philip J. Hilts, 2003

AMERICAN GUIDANCE FOR SENIORS by Ken Skala, 1992

HEALTHY AGING: A Lifelong Guide of Your Physical and Spiritual Well-Being By Andrew Weil, MD 2005

NURISING HOMES & ASSISTED LIVING FACILITIES by Linda H. Connell, 2004

THE 36-HOUR DAY: A Family Guide to Caring for People with Alzheimer Disease, Other Dementias and Memory Loss in Later Life By Nancy L. Mace, MA and Peter V. Robins MD, 2006

LONGEVITY MADE SIMPLE By Richard J. Flanigan MD and Kate Flaningan, MD, MPH, 2007

THE EVERYTHING ALZHEIMER'S BOOK By Carolyn Dean, MD, ND, 2007

ALZHEIMER'S FROM THE INSIDE OUT By Richard Taylor, 2007

ALZHEIMER'S DISEASE: Frequently Asked Questions By Frena Gray-Davidson, 1998

THE ALZHEMER'S ADVISER By Vaughn E. James, 2009

AMERICAN MEDICAL ASSOCIATION

COMPLETE GUIDE TO PREVENTION AND WELLNESS, 2008

About the Author

Eva Mor, PhD, is an epidemiologist and specialist in gerontology and health management. She has worked with the elderly for more than 23 years, in long term facilities, acute hospitals, and facilities for chronic diseases. During her many years in the field she has participated in several planning committees dedicated to issues of the elderly. With a M.A. in Gerontology and Health Management, she has devoted her life to the betterment of the lives of seniors. She currently lives in New York City with her family.